CLINICAL
EPIDEMIOLOGY
–the essentials

CLINICAL EPIDEMIOLOGY
–the essentials

Robert H. Fletcher, M.D., M.Sc.

Associate Professor of Medicine
Clinical Associate Professor of Epidemiology
The University of North Carolina
Chapel Hill, North Carolina

Suzanne W. Fletcher, M.D., M.Sc.

Associate Professor of Medicine
Clinical Associate Professor of Epidemiology
The University of North Carolina
Chapel Hill, North Carolina

Edward H. Wagner, M.D., M.P.H.

Associate Professor
Departments of Medicine and Epidemiology
The University of North Carolina
Chapel Hill, North Carolina

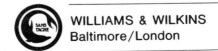

WILLIAMS & WILKINS
Baltimore/London

Made in the United States of America

Reprinted 1983

Library of Congress Cataloging in Publication Data

Fletcher, Robert H.

Clinical epidemiology

    Includes index.
    1.   Epidemiology. 2. Medicine, Clinical. I. Fletcher, Suzanne W. II. Wagner,
Edward. 1940– . III. Title. [DNLM: 1. Epidemiology. WA 105 P614c]
RA652.F55   616   81-21901
ISBN 0-683-03252-6   AACR2

Composed and printed at the
Waverly Press, Inc.
Mt. Royal and Guilford Aves.
Baltimore, MD 21202, U.S.A.

DEDICATION

To the Sydenhams of Medicine—past, present, and future.

PREFACE

"Clinical epidemiology" is a term none of us had heard during our training. But our need for it became apparent when we first took responsibility for patients. During our "basic science" years in medical school the facts in medicine had seemed formidably embodied in physiologic laws, histologic descriptions, and biochemical pathways. When we became involved in the care of patients, however, we found that the clinical world often operated by a very different set of rules. It was more difficult to determine what was true and not true about clinical medicine, and the ways in which that was judged. At the same time knowing the facts, which until then had been a matter of pure intellectual curiosity, became an urgent necessity. Like other conscientious physicians, we wanted to be reasonably certain that we were doing more good than harm by our actions.

Where could the best possible answers to clinical questions be found?

One approach was to apply the basic principles of human biology. Using knowledge of the chemistry, physiology, and anatomy of disease to solve clinical problems was certainly stimulating and often elegant as well. Sometimes it seemed to be just the right way to proceed. But there were many situations in which this approach fell wide of the mark because of substantial conceptual gaps between the structured experience of basic science and the more complex, open-ended problems arising in the care of patients.

Sometimes we were comfortable taking the word of a trusted authority. But the limitations of this approach were apparent. For one thing, experts often disagreed and so could not all be right. Not only did they disagree about the wisdom of a given diagnostic or therapeutic approach, but also about the validity of the evidence upon which their recommendations were based. Also, most faculty were involved in laboratory research and found it difficult to apply the kind of scientific approaches used in the laboratory to the solution of clinical problems. Evidence that could not be reduced to "hard science" was sometimes viewed by them with uncertainty and suspicion. Moreover, it became clear that experts' personalities and self-interest colored their interpretation of clinical data, as they do for all of us.

So we, like many others, felt compelled to make up our own minds about important clinical questions, referring to published research. It was soon apparent that we had received no formal schooling in this subject. We found ourselves floundering through the medical literature, trying to use intuition, common sense, and good judgment. Although it was clear that we had much to learn, it was not clear what we needed to learn, or how to go about it.

For years, epidemiologists had been asking similar questions about disease, and trying to find the best possible ways to answer them. Epidemiologists paid particular attention to how the validity of human research was affected when it was not possible to perform highly structured experiments, as one might in a laboratory. They had this in common with clinical researchers, and so many of the solutions they devised were highly relevant to clinical medicine. But because epidemiologists and clinicians did not have a history of working together, the flow of information between them had been retarded.

We were fortunate to receive formal training in epidemiology as clinicians, and to be exposed to thoughtful physicians who recognized the potential contribution of that discipline to clinical medicine (see Acknowledgments). With them, we began to develop ways to teach clinicians the application of epidemiologic methods and perspectives to the solution of clinical problems.

When we began to teach our clinical epidemiology course to students and housestaff, we found efforts hindered by the absence of a suitable text. Although a rich array of writings about clinical epidemiology were available, they had not been drawn together, summarized, and simplified in a single book. So we, set out to fill this need.

In our book, we have attempted to present the material as simply as possible, and to draw particular attention to major landmarks in a rather cluttered landscape. We recognize that there may be sections in which we have omitted more details than those with a special interest in this field might prefer. We did so for the sake of clarity on the basic issues.

We intend this book for all those who are involved in clinical medicine, and want to examine empirical data on their own, in order to make an independent judgment as to the utility of those data in the care of patients. Potential readers include medical students, housestaff, "fully trained" physicians, nurse practitioners, or others engaged in providing care to patients. Because the authors are internists, many of the clinical examples concern medical problems of adults. However, we do not believe that the audience is limited by clinical specialty or seniority. It is our experience, backed by some published studies, that understanding the principles of clinical epidemiology is not concentrated in one or another specialty, and does not necessarily grow with training and experience—as might, for example, knowledge of the content of the medical literature.

Clinical epidemiology contributes to understanding both observations made by individual clinicians and reports of research done by others. Many clinicians do not anticipate a career in research, and so might wonder if learning about research is worthwhile. It seems to us that researchers who collect clinical data and clinicians who use it have a great deal in common. Both have a critical stake in the accuracy of the information. Researchers may need to know more about the particulars of gathering and analyzing the data, and spend more time at it. But clinicians must understand the basic principles of research in order to interpret what is found.

For these reasons, we believe clinical epidemiology is a basic science for clinicians. We rely on it when patient care begins, the evidence is reviewed, and decisions must be made.

ACKNOWLEDGMENTS

We consider ourselves extremely fortunate to have come of age in medicine during the past two decades. There have been dramatic changes in the kind of information available to clinicians, both "at the bedside" and in the medical literature. It has been stimulating both to have the information, and to participate in efforts to improve the way in which it is gathered and evaluated.

Along the way, we have been influenced by some unusual colleagues. John Cassel and Leon Gordis awakened us to the kinship between classical epidemiology and clinical medicine. Our initial clinical chairmen, Charles Carpenter, Evan Calkins, and John Beck were among the first to welcome physicians with our kind of training and interests into clinical departments of medicine. Alvan Feinstein and David Sackett have pursued the intellectual domain of clinical epidemiology with extraordinary energy and candor. They are largely responsible for its growth. Michel Ibrahim, our present Chairman of Epidemiology, has built bridges between epidemiology and clinical medicine, and created an intellectual environment in which clinical epidemiology could flourish. Our colleagues in the practice of medicine have served to keep us on track by asking the right questions, about real patients, from day to day. These are the students, housestaff, and faculty at our various points along the way, particularly Johns Hopkins, Buffalo, McGill, and the University of North Carolina. We hope this book reflects in some measure both the wisdom of our mentors, and the impatient quest for relevance that has marked our clinical colleagues.

As for the process of writing this book, it has certainly been exhilarating, but at times tedious as well. We have been sustained during the difficult periods by the generosity of a great many colleagues at the University of North Carolina. We are particularly grateful to those who worked with us on the clinical epidemiology course for medical students at McGill and UNC. Several colleagues made special efforts to critique the manuscript, among them Mack Lipkin, Dale Williams, Michel Ibrahim, and fellows in the Robert Wood Johnson Clinical Scholars Program.

The Robert Wood Johnson Clinical Scholars Program has exerted a constant influence on our professional lives. The foresight and hard work of those who developed the Program have helped create an environment in academic medicine which has promoted the growth of clinical epidemiology.

For real work, and critical work at that, our secretaries deserve our greatest thanks. Heidi McMurray, Shelley Gonzales, Rebecca Evans, and Pat Taylor completed many drafts with unfailing accuracy and good will—and without a word processor! Linda Thompson drew most of the figures, and was always patient with our many special requests.

To all of these people, we owe our gratitude. They have made clinical medicine a great deal more fun and meaningful for us.

CONTENTS

Preface vii

Acknowledgments ix

Chapter 1. Introduction   1

Chapter 2. Abnormality 18

Chapter 3. Diagnostic Test 41

Chapter 4. Diagnostic Strategies 59

Chapter 5. Frequency 75

Chapter 6. Risk 91

Chapter 7. Prognosis 106

Chapter 8. Treatment 127

Chapter 9. Chance 153

Chapter 10. Rare Disease 168

Chapter 11. Cause 185

Chapter 12. Summing up 203

Index 219

chapter

1

Introduction

A 52-year-old man is admitted to the hospital because of abdominal pain and weight loss. He was well until 8 weeks prior to admission when he noticed the gradual onset of epigastric pain radiating to the back. Over the next several weeks this pain increased in intensity and became constant. In retrospect, he has had a poor appetite and has lost about 15 pounds in the past few months. He consulted his physician and a diagnostic evaluation, including a complete history, physical examination, a complete blood count, and serum chemistries disclosed no specific cause for his symptoms.

This patient is likely to have many questions. Am I sick? Are you sure? What is causing my sickness? How will it affect me? What can be done about it?

The clinician caring for the patient faces the same set of questions, but at a more sophisticated level. In addition, it is the clinician's task to provide the answers. For instance, the physician must differentiate between carcinoma of the pancreas and peptic ulcer disease, among other possible causes for this patient's complaints. If an upper gastrointestinal series is performed and it is reported to be "normal", the doctor must have some idea of how frequently a "false negative" result can occur in the presence of these diseases, and must decide if further testing is warranted. If a subsequent abdominal computerized tomography scan shows a pancreatic mass and a diagnosis of pancreatic cancer is made, the patient will probably want to know the prognosis of pancreatic cancer—how long such patients live and how well they fare. Finally, the

1

physician must decide which kinds of treatment—surgery, chemotherapy, or simple palliative care—offer the most help to the patient.

As clinicians, we use various means to find answers to these types of questions. Most of all, we rely on our own experiences, the experiences of our colleagues, and the medical literature. In short, we depend on past observations made on other patients. The manner with which such observations are made frequently determines whether the clinical conclusions we reach are valid.

Table 1.1
Clinical Issues and Questions in the Practice of Medicine

Issue	Question
Normality/Abnormality	Is a person sick or well?
	What abnormalities are associated with having a disease?
Diagnosis	How accurate are diagnostic tests or strategies used to find a disease?
Frequency	How often does a disease occur?
Risk	What factors are associated with an increased likelihood of disease?
Prognosis	What are the consequences of having a disease?
Treatment	How does treatment change the future course of a disease?
Cause	What conditions result in disease?
	What is the pathogenetic mechanism of disease?

CLINICAL EPIDEMIOLOGY

Clinical epidemiology is one approach to making and interpreting scientific observations in medicine. *Clinical epidemiology* is the application of epidemiologic principles and methods to problems encountered in clinical medicine. It is a science concerned with counting clinical events occurring in intact human beings, and it uses epidemiologic methods to carry out and analyze the count.

Types of questions addressed by clinical epidemiology are listed in Table 1.1. By and large, these are the same questions confronting the doctor and patient in the example presented at the beginning of this chapter. They are at issue in most doctor-patient encounters.

The clinical events of primary interest in clinical epidemiology are the health outcomes of particular concern to patients and those caring for them (Table 1.2). They are the "dependent variables" in medical practice, because they are the events doctors try to change when treating patients.

Thus, an important distinction between clinical epidemiology and other sciences contributing to medicine is that the events of interest in clinical epidemiology can be studied directly only in intact humans and not in animals or pieces of humans such as tissue cultures, pituitary hormones, or red cell membranes.

The methods used to count the clinical events were developed primarily in the field of epidemiology, which has been defined as "the study of the distribution and determinants of disease frequency in man" (1). These methods are the subject of this book.

Table 1.2
Health Outcomes and Clinical Events (The Five D's)*

Health Outcome	Clinical Events and Relevance
Death	A universal health outcome, the timeliness of the event being the issue.
Disease	A combination of symptoms, physical signs and laboratory test results.
Disability	The functional status of patients in terms of ability to live independently and go about their daily lives at home, work, or recreation.
Discomfort	Uncomfortable symptoms such as pain, nausea, vertigo, tinnitis, or fatigue.
Dissatisfaction	Emotional and mental states such as agitation, sadness, or anger.

* Some suggest a sixth "D"—destitution—because physicians should be concerned with financial consequences of health care to their patients. Others have pointed out that the five D's emphasize the negative side of health outcomes. Nevertheless, the five D's do remind physicians that clinical events other than death and disease are important.

The basic purpose of clinical epidemiology is to develop and apply methods of clinical observation which will lead to valid clinical conclusions. For clinicians who intend to make up their own minds about the soundness of clinical information, some understanding of this field is as necessary as an understanding of anatomy, pathology, biochemistry, and pharmacology. Indeed, clinical epidemiology is one of the basic sciences forming the foundation on which modern medicine is practiced.

Even so, the principles of clinical epidemiology are not yet second nature to most clinicians. This is partly related to underlying differences between the parent disciplines, clinical medicine and epidemiology. Both are scientific approaches to the causes and consequences of disease in humans. Both have a practical bent, by and large seeking to discover information that can be useful in the control of disease and alleviation of suffering. However, there are some rather stark differences between them as well. When we have explored these differences, we will consider how they can be brought together for the purpose of enriching our understanding of clinical medicine.

Clinical Medicine

As most readers of this book know, clinicians are, by and large, concerned with individual patients. They meet all of their patients personally, take their own histories, and do their own physical examinations. Usually they are not interested in how patients happen to be found in their practices, as opposed to some other medical setting. As a result, clinicians usually do not feel particularly responsible for other patients, who may be just as sick but have not come to their attention. Their work is guided by their experience in the specific health care settings in which they practice, and not by experience with the population at large.

Clinicians bear intense personal responsibility for individual patients. Therefore, they tend to see what is special about each patient. Thus, it is not surprising that clinicians are often reluctant to lump patients into crude categories of risk, diagnosis, or treatment. Many have a distinct uneasiness about uncertainty, and the ways it is expressed through probabilities.

Clinical training is largely oriented towards the mechanisms of disease through study of biochemistry, anatomy, physiology, and other basic sciences. These traditional basic sciences are powerful influences in a a medical student's formative years, and go on to become the predominant forces in clinical research and publications. This fosters the belief that to understand medicine is to understand the detailed processes of disease in individual patients. The implication is that one can predict the course of disease and develop treatments through knowledge of its mechanisms.

Epidemiology

Epidemiology is the research discipline concerned with the distribution and determinants of disease in populations. Epidemiologists differ from clinicians in several ways. Compared to clinicians, epidemiologists are more concerned that their observations are representative of some defined group of people, or "population." They wish to record the experiences of all members of the group, whether or not they are sick, and whether or not they have come to medical attention. Epidemiologists usually do not personally collect all their data themselves nor do they usually meet the people they study. Because they work with groups rather than with individual patients, epidemiologists must accept uncertainty. Perhaps it is easier for them to do so because they do not have a personal stake in the individual subjects they study.

When epidemiologists study disease, their categories are often crude by clinical standards. They work with such variables as "smokers" and "non-smokers", or "sudden death" and "myocardial infarction", even though a myriad of special circumstances are hidden within these classes.

Epidemiologists are generally more interested in whether something occurs than in how it occurs at a pathogenetic, mechanistic level. They rely in part on an understanding of the mechanism of disease to form hypotheses, and then test these hypotheses in human populations. However, if a pathogenetic mechanism is not known, epidemiologists do not necessarily discard a hypothesis. For example, if it can be shown that cigarette smoking in itself is related to cardiovascular disease, and the risk of heart disease decreases when smoking ceases, everything else being equal, the epidemiologist might consider the role of smoking in heart disease largely settled. The more mechanistically inclined clinical researcher might remain quite dissatisfied until the causative agent in cigarette smoke is isolated, and the pathway by which it causes heart disease is laid out.

Because epidemiologists work with groups of individuals, each of which displays unique genetic and environmental characteristics, their stock-in-trade is to know how to deal with unwanted variables in human research. Along the way, they work closely with biostatisticians, who use statistics to summarize the experience of groups, adjust for unwanted differences between groups being compared, and assess whether chance could have determined the findings.

Clinical Epidemiology

As both clinicians and epidemiologists have become increasingly aware that their fields interrelate, clinical epidemiology has begun to develop. It has been proposed as a distinct discipline within medicine in recognition of the following:

1. Many clinical decisions are based on information which is uncertain and, therefore, expressed as a probability.

2. That probability is best estimated by means of past experience with similar patients.

3. Because clinical observations are made on subjects who are free to do as they please, by clinicians with variable skills and prejudices, the observations may be influenced by a variety of systematic errors which can distort the true nature of events and thereby be misleading.

4. To deal with these misleading effects, clinical observations should be based on sound scientific principles, which requires an understanding of the design of human research.

5. Because clinical observations also can be influenced by the play of chance, interpretation of the observations requires an understanding of statistics.

6. Understanding these principles is as important to clinicians who wish to be self-sufficient in judging clinical information as it is to researchers who will produce research.

7. Although the principles of clinical scientific methods are implicit in a great deal of current clinical teaching, they are not a formal part of most medical curricula.

A growing understanding of the relevance of epidemiology to clinical medicine is reflected in the recent development of clinical epidemiology

'ical students, the increased numbers of articles in clinical
ˌ with precepts of clinical epidemiology, and the develop-
ˌˌowship programs for training clinicians in clinical epidemiol-

We hope this book will contribute to the growth of clinical epidemiology by bringing together, in a few pages, the essentials of epidemiology that are important to the clinician's world. We also hope that this book will help clinicians evaluate the constant flow of new medical information. This means clinicians must learn about the various research designs used in medical research and something about the strengths and pitfalls of these various designs. With such knowledge, conscientious clinicians can develop skills which will help them decide whether new information is worthy of the effort to master it in the first place. For those of us with limited, already oversaturated medical memories, such a skill is indeed useful.

Table 1.3
Possible Explanations for Clinical Observations

BIAS
> The observation is incorrect because a systematic error was introduced by:
> Selection bias—the method by which patients were selected for observation.
> Measurement bias—the method by which the observation or measurement was made.
> Confounding bias—the presence of another variable which accounts for the observation.

CHANCE
> The observation is incorrect because of error arising from random variation.

TRUTH
> The observation is correct. (Accept this explanation only after excluding the others!)

BASIC PRINCIPLES

As stated earlier, the basic purpose of clinical epidemiology is to foster methods of clinical observations and interpretation which will lead to valid conclusions. Whenever a clinical question is answered by observing human beings, there are three possible explanations for the answer (Table 1.3). The observation may be incorrect because of bias or chance, or it may be correct.

Bias

Bias is a systematic error in measurement, or a systematic difference (other than the one of interest), between groups. For example, when Treatment A seems to work better than Treatment B, but A is given to healthier patients than B, the results could be due to the systematic difference in health between the groups of patients rather than to differences in treatment. Or A might taste better than B so that patients take the drug more regularly. Or A might be a new, highly popular drug and B an old drug, so that researchers and patients might be more inclined to think that the new drug works better. All of these situations are examples of the potential for bias.

Compared to basic science research, observations on patients (whether for patient care or research) are particularly prone to bias. Such observations tend to be just plain untidy. As subjects under study, human beings have the disconcerting habit of doing as they please and not necessarily what would be required for scientific rigor. When one attempts to conduct an experiment with them, as one might in a laboratory, things tend to go wrong. Some refuse to participate whereas others drop out or choose another treatment. What is more, some of the most important things about humans—feelings, comfort, performance—are generally more difficult to measure than physical properties like blood pressure or serum sodium. The methods of measuring and determining whether instruments used to measure these events are properly designed and tested are less direct. Then, too, there is the normal inclination of clinicians to see that their therapies succeed. (Most patients would not want a physician who felt otherwise.) This attitude, so important in the practice of medicine, makes clinical observations particularly vulnerable to bias.

Although dozens of particular biases have been defined, most biases which threaten the validity of clinical observations fall into one of three broad categories (and are covered in detail in succeeding chapters):

1. *Selection bias* occurs when observations are made on a group of patients that has been assembled incorrectly

Example—A study showed an association between the antihypertensive agent, reserpine, and breast cancer in women (2). In the study, reserpine use among a group of women with breast cancer was compared to reserpine use among a group of women without breast cancer. However, women without breast cancer whose first discharge diagnosis was a cardiovascular diagnosis (frequently associated with hypertension), were excluded from the study. The results of the study, showing a relationship between reserpine and breast cancer, may have been due to avoiding this potential bias, found no association whereby women without breast cancer but likely to be on reserpine were systematically excluded from the study. Other studies of the question, avoiding this selection bias, found no association between reserpine and breast cancer (3).

2. *Measurement bias* occurs when the methods of measurement are consistently dissimilar among groups of patients

An example of a potential measurement bias would be in the use of information taken from medical records to determine if women on birth control pills were more at risk for thromboembolism than those not on "the pill." Suppose a study were made comparing the frequency of oral contraceptive use among women admitted to a hospital because of thrombophlebitis and a group of women admitted for other reasons. It is entirely possible that housestaff, aware of the reported association between estrogens and thrombotic events would obtain and record information about oral contraceptive use more thoroughly for women with phlebitis than for those without phlebitis. If so, an observed association between oral contraceptives and thrombophlebitis could be due to the biased way in which the medical histories were obtained and recorded.

3. *Confounding bias* occurs when two factors or processes are interrelated, or "travel together", and it is incorrectly concluded that one of the factors is the causal agent

Example—Several studies have shown that serum triglyceride levels (TG) are associated with risk for coronary heart disease (CHD): the higher the TG, the higher the risk. Because of this, clinicians have screened for TG and attempted to lower TG when it was elevated. This might be helpful if TG were an independent cause of CHD. But other known causes of CHD, particularly elevated serum cholesterol levels and reduced levels of high density lipoprotein are related both to serum triglycerides and CHD. When the contribution of these other factors is held constant, using a statistical technique, the relationship between TG and CHD no longer is present. It seems unlikely therefore that TG is an independent cause of CHD; its apparent relationship to CHD is confounded with other factors which are independent causes (4).

It should be apparent that selection bias and confounding bias are not mutually exclusive. They are described separately, however, because they present problems at different points in a clinical observation or study. Selection bias is at issue primarily when patients are chosen for observation, and so it is important in the design of a study. Confounding bias comes to the fore in analysis of the data, once the observations have been made.

Usually more than one bias operates at once, as in the following hypothetical example.

Example—A study was done to determine whether regular exercise lowers the risk of CHD. An exercise program was offered to employees of a plant and the rate of subsequent coronary events was compared among employees who volunteered for the program, and those who did not volunteer. Coronary events were determined by means of regular voluntary check-ups, including a careful history and electrocardiogram, as well as routine health records. The group that exercised had lower rates of CHD. However, they also smoked cigarettes less.

In this example, selection bias could be present if volunteers taking the exercise program were, for some reason, at lower risk for coronary disease even before the program began—e.g., because they had lower serum lipids or less family history of coronary disease. Measurement bias might have occurred because the exercise group stood a better chance of having a coronary event detected, inasmuch as more of them were likely to be examined routinely. Finally, the conclusion that exercise lowered the risk of coronary disease might be the result of a confounding bias if the association between exercise and coronary events in this particular study resulted from the fact that smoking cigarettes is a risk factor for coronary disease and the exercise group smoked less.

From the beginning of the National Institutes of Health era, in the

1950's, many clinical investigators have avoided problems of bias because their work has been in biomedical laboratories. Those questions which could not be answered in the laboratories were labelled the "art of medicine" since they involved so many seemingly uncontrollable variables. Epidemiologists, on the other hand, had no place to retreat. They began tackling the biases, identifying them, cataloging them, and developing strategies to overcome them. The progress made in this area in the past couple of decades has helped give rise to clinical epidemiology.

Chance

A single set of clinical observations may misrepresent the truth because of error arising from random variation. Observations about disease are ordinarily made on a sample of patients rather than all those with the disease in question. Even if a sample is unbiased, actual observations on a single sample are unlikely to correspond exactly to the true state of affairs in the larger group of all patients. However, if the observations were repeated on many such samples, they would be found to vary about the true value. The divergence of an observation on a sample from the true population value, due to chance alone, is called *random variation.*

We are all familiar with chance as an explanation for why a coin does not come up heads exactly 50% of the time when it is flipped, say, 100 times. The same influence of random variation applies when assessing the effects of Treatments A and B, discussed earlier. Suppose all biases were removed from a study of the relative effects of two treatments. Suppose, further, that the two treatments were, in reality, equally effective, each improving about 50% of the patients treated. Even so, because of chance alone, a single study involving small numbers of patients in each treatment group might easily find A improving 80% of the patients and B only 20%.

Chance can affect all steps necessary in making clinical observations. In the assessment of treatments A and B, random variation can occur in the selection of patients for the study, the allocation of patients to the two treatment groups, and the measurements made on the groups.

Unlike bias, which deflects values in one direction or another, random variation is as likely to result in observations above the true value as below. As a consequence, the mean of many unbiased observations on samples tends to correspond to the true value in the population, even though the results of individual small samples may not.

Statistics help estimate the probability of chance or random variation accounting for clinical results. A knowledge of statistics can also help reduce that probability. It is important, however, to understand that random variation cannot be totally eliminated. Chance should always be considered when assessing the results of clinical observations.

Relationship between Bias and Chance

The relationship between bias and chance is illustrated in Figure 1.1. The measurement of diastolic blood pressure on a single patient is taken as an example. True blood pressure can be obtained by an intra-arterial cannula, and multiple readings are illustrated as all being 80 mm Hg. But this method is not possible for routine measurements. Blood pressure is ordinarily measured indirectly, using a sphygmomanometer. The simpler instrument is prone to error, or deviations from the true value. In the example, this is represented by all the sphygmomanometer readings falling to the right of the true value. The deviation of sphygmomanometer readings to the right (bias) may have several explanations: e.g., a poorly calibrated sphygmomanometer, wrong cuff size, or a deaf clinician. Bias could also result if different sounds are chosen to represent diastolic blood pressure. The usual end points—phase IV and phase V Korotkoff sounds—tend to be above and below the true diastolic pressure, respectively; and even that is unpredictable in obese people. If bias were eliminated, individual blood pressure readings would still be subject to error because of random variation in measurement, as illustrated by the spread of the sphygmomanometer readings around the mean value (90 mm Hg).

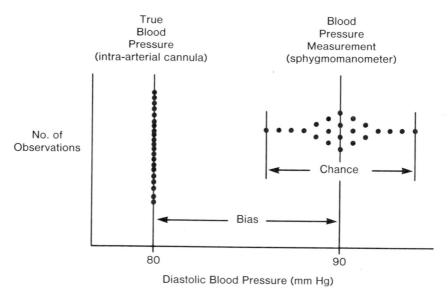

Figure 1.1.   Relationship between Bias and Chance: Blood Pressure Measurements by Intra-Arterial Cannula and Sphygmomanometer.

The two sources of error—bias and chance—are not mutually exclusive. In most situations, both are represented. The main reason for distinguishing between the two is that they are handled differently.

Bias, in theory, can be prevented by conducting clinical observations properly or corrected through proper data analysis. If not eliminated, bias often can be detected by the discerning reader. Most of this book is about how to recognize, avoid, or minimize bias.

Chance cannot be eliminated, but its influence can be reduced by proper design of research, and the remaining error estimated by statistics. Statistics can also help remove the effects of known biases. However, no amount of statistical treatment can correct for unknown biases in data. Some would go so far as to prefer that statistics not be applied to data vulnerable to bias because of poor research design, for fear of giving false respectability to misleading work.

Validity

A clinical observation is valid if it corresponds to the true state of affairs. For the observation to be valid, it must be neither biased nor incorrect due to chance. It is useful to distinguish between two general kinds of validity—internal validity and external validity, or generalizability.

Internal validity is the degree to which the results of an observation are correct for the patients being studied. It is "internal" because it applies to the particular conditions of the particular group of patients being observed, and not necessarily to others. The internal validity of clinical observations is determined by how well they are carried out, and is threatened by all the biases and random variation discussed previously. For a clinical observation to be useful, internal validity is a necessary but often insufficient condition.

Generalizability (external validity) is the degree to which the results of an observation hold true in other settings. For an individual physician, it is an answer to the question: "Assuming the results of a study are true, do they apply to my patient as well?" Generalizability expresses the validity of assuming that patients in a study are comparable to other patients.

An unimpeachable study, with high internal validity, may be totally misleading when the results are generalized to certain other patients. This is because of yet another bias, sampling bias. *Sampling bias occurs when observations and conclusions about one group of patients are generalized to other groups of patients who are not similar.*

Example—Sampling bias was recently demonstrated in studies of febrile seizures in children. Because febrile seizures commonly occur in childhood (reportedly in 2–4% of all children) it is important to know if such seizures recur. If they frequently recur, treatment with anticonvulsant therapy may be worth considering. On the other hand, if febrile seizures are usually one-time phenomena, reassurance of the parents is in order.

Figure 1.2 shows the recurrence rates of seizures among children reported in various studies, according to how the children were chosen for the study. On the *left*, the population-based studies followed up all children in defined population groups who had febrile seizures. The recurrence rates reported in these studies were all very low. Clinic-based studies, shown on the *right* of Figure 1.2, described recurrence rates in children attending hospital clinics or specialty referral units, and were associated with much higher recurrence rates.

Applying the results of referral hospital studies to community practices would result in falsely high estimates of the likelihood of recurring seizures. On the other hand, using the conclusion of the population-based studies when discussing the prognosis of febrile seizures with the parents of a child referred to a pediatric neurology unit might likewise be inaccurate, this time in the opposite direction (5).

Because most clinical studies take place in medical centers and because patients in such centers usually overrepresent the serious end of the disease spectrum, sampling bias in clinical research tends to exaggerate the serious nature of disease.

It should be noted that many authors refer to sampling bias as a selection bias. We prefer to distinguish this "external bias" from the selection bias that threatens internal validity of clinical observations, discussed earlier. Figure 1.3 indicates that selection, measurement, and confounding biases threaten the internal validity of a clinical observation, whereas sampling bias relates to the generalizability of the observation.

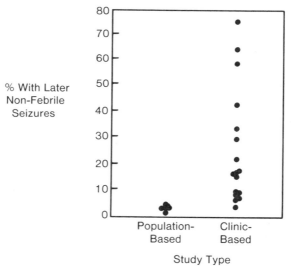

Figure 1.2. Example of Potential Sampling Bias: Recurrent Seizures in Infants with Febrile Seizures in Population-based and Clinic-based Studies. (Redrawn from Ellenberg JH and Nelson KB. *JAMA*, 1980; 243:1337–1340.)

In theory, internal validity and generalizability can both be maximized by proper research design and execution. But in practice, internal validity is easier to achieve than generalizability. As a result, the generalizability of clinical observations, even those that are well made, frequently becomes a matter of opinion about which reasonable people might disagree. For example, the Veterans Administration (VA) study of hypertension treatment was carried out with special attention to potential biases and chance. As a result, the internal validity of this study, with its conclusion that lowering blood pressure decreased risk of death and severe morbid events in the particular patients in the study, is generally accepted (6).

But the study was confined to men. Some clinicians were willing to use the results of this study to guide decisions about treatment of women. Others, more skeptical because of known differences in the frequency of cardiovascular disease between men and women, were unwilling to do so. The VA study itself held no solution to this disagreement. The only way to resolve the dispute was to collect data on women with hypertension. Such studies have subsequently been done and found similar results for women.

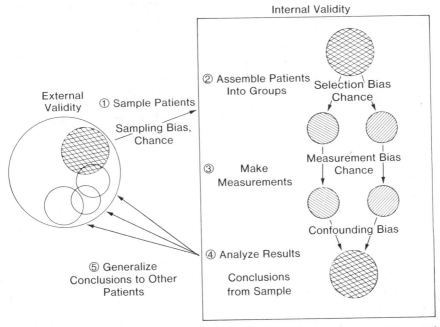

Figure 1.3.   Relationships Among Internal and External Validity, Bias, and Chance.

METHODS AND CONCLUSIONS

A basic tenet of this book is that good methods of clinical observation lead to correct conclusions, i.e., observations which are relatively free of systematic error (bias) and which cannot be easily discounted as arising from chance alone are likely to be correct. A skeptic might ask: what reason have we for believing that such methods lead to correct conclusions?

First, there is often a systematic relationship between the strength of research methods and the findings. An example is shown in Table 1.4. For many years there has been controversy over the effectiveness of Bacille Calmette Guérin vaccine in preventing active tuberculosis. Study results have varied from a reported 80% of cases being prevented by the vaccine, to the other extreme in which vaccinated persons have 56% more tuberculosis! Various biologic explanations have been advanced to account for these results, including differences among studies in the strength of the vaccine, the susceptibility of the subjects, and the extent of their exposure to tuberculosis. Recently, the methods of these studies have been subjected to rigorous scrutiny. It was found that the reported effectiveness of the vaccine was greatest in studies which met basic criteria for good methods, and least in studies which did not. Other reviews have also found a systematic relationship between methods and conclusions, including reviews of anticoagulants for acute myocardial infarction (7), corticosteroids for gram negative sepsis (8), and coronary bypass surgery and death (9).

Second, conclusions from studies with relatively sound methods have been less readily refuted by subsequent observations. In the 1950's, it was supposed that implanting the mammary artery into the myocardium would relieve angina pectoris and prevent mortality by reestablishing coronary circulation. Reports of experience with the operation, which were not methodologically sound, attested to its value. However, it was

Table 1.4

Relationship Between Strength of Study Methods and Results: Bacille Calmette Guérin (BCG) Immunization Against Tuberculosis*

Strength of Study Methods	Number of Studies	BCG Protection (%)
Strong	3	75 to 80
Weak	5	−56 to 29

* From Clemens J.D. *Clin Res* 1981; 29:499A.

later shown that the implanted arteries usually were not patent, or did not anastomose freely with the coronary circulation, even in patients who had experienced relief of pain. Therefore, the only plausible reason why the operation might work, at least on a physiologic basis, was not supported. On the other hand, the value of coronary bypass surgery for prevention of death in specific subgroups of patients has been established by carefully performed clinical trials.

INFORMATION AND DECISIONS

The primary concern of this book is the quality of information and its correct interpretation in making clinical decisions. Making decisions are another matter. True, good decisions depend on good information; but they involve a great deal more as well, including value judgments and the weighing of competing risks and benefits.

In recent years, a variety of methods for "quantitative" decision-making have become popular. Among these are decision analysis, cost-benefit analysis, and cost-effectiveness analysis. They involve presenting the decision-making process in an explicit way, so that the components of the decision, and the consequences of assigning various values to them can be examined. Some aspects of decision analysis, such as evaluation of diagnostic tests, are included in this book. However, we have elected not to go deeply into decision analysis itself. Our justification is that ultimately decisions are only as good as the information used to make them, and we have found enough to say about the essentials of collecting and interpreting clinical information to fill a book. Readers who wish to delve deeper into decision analysis can begin with some of the readings suggested at the end of this chapter.

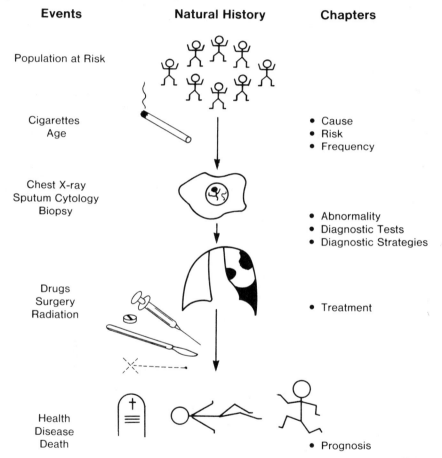

Figure 1.4.   Organization of Book, Illustrated for the Disease, Lung Cancer. Issues Covered in Chapters on Chance, Cause, and Rare Diseases Relate to the Entire Progression of Disease.

ORGANIZATION OF BOOK

In most text books of clinical medicine, information about disease is presented as answers to traditional clinical questions, as outlined in Table 1.1. On the other hand, most books about clinical investigation are organized around research strategies: clinical trials, surveys, case-control studies, etc. This way of organizing a book may serve those who would perform clinical research, but it is often awkward for clinicians. As a result, clinicians do not have a comprehensive source of information about the basic structure of clinical observations as it relates to clinical practice, as they do for the clinical relevance of the basic sciences. For example, none of the over 800 books and journals in "A Library for Internists", recommended by the American College of Physicians, is about the methods of clinical observation per se (10).

This book is written for clinicians who wish to understand the methods of clinical observation and research. We have not written primarily for those who would perform clinical research, but for all the rest who depend on it. However, we believe that the basic needs of those who create and those who use clinical research findings are similar.

We have organized the book primarily according to the clinical questions surrounding doctor-patient encounters. Figure 1.4 illustrates how these questions correspond to the book chapters, taking as an example the disease, lung cancer. The questions relate to the entire natural history of disease, from the time non-diseased people are first exposed to risk, through when some acquire the disease and emerge as patients, until the end results of disease are manifest.

In each chapter, the clinical epidemiologic strategies used to answer the clinical questions are described. Occasionally, a given strategy, such as a cohort study, may be useful in answering several clinical questions. For the purposes of presentation, we have arbitrarily discussed these strategies primarily in one chapter. But is is important to keep in mind that given clinical epidemiologic methods may be applicable to more than one clinical question. When this is so, we have attempted to refer to these methods in other relevant chapters.

Suggested Readings

Feinstein AR. Why clinical epidemiology? *Clin Res*, 1972; 20:821–825.
Sackett DL. Clinical epidemiology. *Am J Epid*, 1969; 89:125–128.
Feinstein AR. Clinical Judgment. Baltimore: The Williams & Wilkins Company, 1967.
Department of Clinical Epidemiology and Biostatistics, McMaster University Health Sciences Centre. Clinical Epidemiology Rounds. How to read clinical journals I–IV. *Can Med Assoc J*, 1981; 124:555–558, 703–710, 869–872, 985–990, 1156–1162.
Feinstein AR. Clinical Biostatistics. St. Louis: CV Mosby Co., 1977.
Murphy EA. The Logic of Medicine. Baltimore: The Johns Hopkins University Press, 1976.
Wulff HR. Rational Diagnosis and Treatment. Oxford: Blackwell Scientific Publications, 1976.
Weinstein MC, Fineberg HV, Elstein AS, Fraizer HS, Neuhauser D, Neutra RR, McNeil BJ. Clinical Decision Analysis. Philadelphia: WB Saunders, 1980.
McNeil BJ, Keeler E, Adelstein SJ. Primer on certain elements of medical decision making. *N Engl J Med*, 1975; 293:211–215.
Riegelman RK. Studying a Study and Testing a Test. How to Read the Medical Literature. Boston: Little, Brown & Co., 1981.
Gehlbach SH. Interpreting the Medical Literature. A Clinician's Guide. Lexington, MA: D. C. Heath and Co., 1982.

References

1. MacMahon B, Pugh TF. Epidemiology. Principles and Methods. Boston: Little, Brown, and Company, 1970.
2. Boston Collaborative Drug Surveillance Program: Reserpine and breast cancer. *Lancet*, 1974; 2:669–671.
3. Ibrahim MA (Ed). The Case Control Study. Consensus and controversy. Elmsford, New York: Pergamon Press, 1979.
4. Hulley SB, Rosenman RH, Bawol RD, Brand RJ. Epidemiology as a guide to clinical decisions: The association between triglyceride and coronary heart disease. *N Engl J Med*, 1980; 302:1383–1389.
5. Ellenberg JH, Nelson KB. Sample selection and the natural history of disease: Studies of febrile seizures. *JAMA*, 1980; 243:1337–1340.
6. Veterans Administration Cooperative Study Group on Antihypertensive Agents. Effects of treatment on morbidity in hypertension. *JAMA*, 1967; 202:1028–1034 and 1970; 213:1143–1152.
7. Gifford RH, Feinstein AR. A critique of methodology in studies of anticoagulant therapy for acute myocardial infarction. *N Engl J Med*, 1969; 280:351–357.
8. Weitzman S, Berger S. Clinical trial design in studies of corticosteroids for bacterial infections. *Ann Intern Med*, 1974; 81:36–42.
9. American Federation for Clinical Research. The scientific uses and abuses of the clinical trial: Treatment of chronic stable angina with saphenous vein bypass grafting. Randomized Veterans Administration Cooperative Study. *Clin Res*, 1978; 26:229–235.
10. Allyn R. A library for internists III. Recommended by the American College of Physicians. *Ann Intern Med*, 1979; 90:446–477.

chapter

2

Abnormality

Clinicians spend a great deal of time distinguishing "normal" from "abnormal" biology. When confronted with something grossly different from the usual, there is of course little difficulty telling the two apart. We are all familiar with pictures in classic textbooks of physical diagnosis showing obvious, even grotesque, examples of massive hepatosplenomegaly, goiter, or elephantiasis. We need take no particular pride in recognizing this kind of abnormality. More often, however, subtler distinctions must be made. Is fleeting chest pain pleurisy or inconsequential? Is a soft systolic heart sound a sign of valvular heart disease or an innocent murmur? Is a slightly elevated serum alkaline phosphatase evidence for liver disease, asymptomatic Paget's disease, or nothing at all?

Decisions about what is abnormal are at their most difficult among unselected, usually ambulatory patients. When patients have already been screened and selected for special attention, as is the case in most referral centers, it is usually clear that something is wrong. The task is then to refine a description of the problem and treat it. In primary care settings, however, subtle manifestations of disease are freely mixed with more everyday complaints, and it is not possible to pursue all of those complaints aggressively. Which of many patients with abdominal pain have self-limited gastroenteritis and which has early appendicitis? Which patients with sore throat and hoarseness have a "garden variety" pharyngitis and which the rare but potentially lethal hemophilus epiglottitis?

These are examples of how difficult, and important, distinguishing various kinds of abnormality can be.

The point of distinguishing normal from abnormal is to separate out those observations which should be considered for action from those which can be discounted. Clinically, observations considered normal are usually described as "within normal limits", "unremarkable", or "noncontributory", and remain buried in the body of a medical history. The abnormal are set out under a problem list, "impressions" or "diagnoses" and are the basis for action.

Simply calling clinical findings normal or abnormal is undoubtedly crude, and results in some misclassification. The justification for taking this approach is that there are times when it is impractical, or unnecessary, to consider the raw data in all their detail. As Bertrand Russell put

Table 2.1

Summarization of Clinical Data. A Patient's Problem List and the Data on which it is Based

Problem List	Raw Data
1. Hypertension	Several blood pressure readings: 170/102, 150/85, 165/92, 173/96
2. Diabetes Mellitus	Glucose tolerance test Time (hours) 0 ½ 1 2 Plasma glu- 110 190 170 140 cose (mg/100 ml)
3. Renal Insufficiency	Serum chemistries: Creatinine 2.7 mg/100 ml Urea nitrogen 40 mg/100 ml Bicarbonate 18 mEq/liter

it, "to be perfectly intelligible one must be inaccurate, and to perfectly accurate, one must be unintelligible." Physicians usually choose to err on the side of being intelligible—to themselves and others—even at the expense of some accuracy. Another reason for simplifying data is that each aspect of a physician's work ends in a decision: to pursue evaluation or to wait; to select a treatment, reassure, or caution. Under these circumstances some sort of classification becomes necessary.

Table 2.1 is an example of how relatively simplistic expressions of abnormality are derived from more complex clinical data. On the *left* is a typical problem list, serving as a statement of the patient's important medical problems. On the *right* are some of the data upon which the decisions to call them problems are based. Conclusions from the data, represented by the problem list, are by no means non-controversial. The mean of the four diastolic blood pressure measurements is 94 mm Hg. Some might argue that this level of blood pressure does not justify the label "hypertension", because it is not particularly high and there are some disadvantages to telling patients they are sick and giving them pills. Others might consider the label fair, considering that this level of blood pressure is associated with an increased risk of cardiovascular disease, and that the risk can be reduced by treatment. The decision to include "diabetes mellitus" is similarly controversial, because the patient's glucose intolerance meets old criteria for diabetes but does not meet recent criteria. Nevertheless, the list serves as a basis for actions—diagnosis, prognosis, treatment—and decisions have to be made, whether actively or passively.

This chapter will present some of the ways clinicians distinguish normal from abnormal. In order to do so, first it will be necessary to consider how biologic observations are measured, expressed, and distributed among unselected people. Then it will be possible to consider how these data are used as a basis for value judgments about what is worth calling abnormal. It will be seen that a variety of approaches to abnormality are used, to suit the situation.

CLINICAL MEASUREMENT

There are three principal scales used for measuring clinical phenomena: nominal, ordinal, and interval.

Data which can only be placed into categories, without any inherent order, are called *nominal*. Relatively few clinical phenomena can be categorized with such sharp distinction that they might be considered truly nominal. Most of these phenomena are determined by a small set of genes (e.g., tissue antigens, sex, inborn errors of metabolism) or are dramatic, discrete events (e.g., death, dialysis, or surgery). Data like these can be placed in categories without much concern about misclassification. It only remains to determine the clinical significance of belonging to one of the categories.

On the other hand, the great majority of clinical data possess some inherent ordering of values: small to large, good to bad, etc. For some data, the order is known but the size of the intervals between values is not. Data which are ordered, but for which the size of the intervals cannot be specified, are called *ordinal* data. Some clinical examples include: mild-moderate-severe dyspnea, and 1+ to 4+ leg edema.

Interval data are both ordered, and represented by intervals of known size.* These include counts like heart rate or seizures per year, which are expressed as integers, as well as measurements like centimeters, milligrams, or milliequivalents for which values fall on a continuum, and the size of intervals is determined by the precision of instruments used to make the measurements.

It is for ordinal and interval data that the question arises: where does

---

* Strictly speaking, if there is a clearly understood zero point such scales have been called "ratio" rather than interval.

normal leave off and abnormal begin? When, for example, does a large normal prostate become too large to be considered normal? Although we are free to chose any cut-off point, usually there are good reasons for our choice. Some of these reasons will be considered later in this chapter.

"HARD" AND "SOFT" MEASUREMENTS

Although evaluation of symptoms plays a major role in clinical medicine, ways of measuring symptoms have received relatively little attention in the medical literature. Often, physical measurement is considered the science and non-physical assessment the art of medicine. This has had, in our opinion, the effect of distorting the "picture" of medicine presented by published research.

As Feinstein puts it:

The term "hard" is usually applied to data that are reliable and preferably dimensional (e.g., laboratory data, demographic data, and financial costs). But clinical performance, convenience, anticipation, and familial data are "soft." They depend on subjective statements, usually expressed in words rather than numbers, by the people who are the observers and the observed.

To avoid such soft data, the results of treatment are commonly restricted to laboratory information that can be objective, dimensional and reliable—but it is also dehumanized. If we are told that the serum cholesterol is 230 mg per 100 ml, that the chest X-ray shows cardiac enlargement, and that the electrocardiogram has Q waves, we would not know whether the treated object was a dog or a person. If we were told that capacity at work was restored, that the medicine tasted good and was easy to take, and that the family was happy about the results, we would recognize a human set of responses.

With suitable attention given to the scientific challenges, the quality of soft data could be hardened (1).

"Soft" phenomena—like pain, anxiety, and nausea—can be measured using methods developed in the social sciences. Most clinicians are simply not familiar with these methods, because of the emphasis medical education places on the hard sciences. By selection and training physicians value the kind of precise measurements the physical and biological sciences afford. Sometimes, however, this approach is at the expense of clinical relevance.

VALIDITY AND RELIABILITY

Two concepts are used to describe the quality of measurements, regardless of the scale on which they are expressed. These concepts are called validity and reliability.

Validity

As pointed out in Chapter 1, *validity* is the degree to which the results of a measurement correspond to the true state of affairs. Another word for validity is accuracy.

For clinical observations that can be measured by physical means, it is relatively easy to establish validity. The observed measurement is compared to some accepted standard. For example, serum sodium can be measured on an instrument recently calibrated against solutions made up with known concentrations of sodium. Similarly, the validity of a physical finding can be established by the results of surgery or an autopsy.

For other clinical measurements, however, no physical standards of validity exist. Among these are pain, nausea, dyspnea, anxiety, and fear. For these, it is necessary to turn to instruments like questionnaires, rather than machines. It is also necessary to use less direct ways of establishing validity. For a questionnaire about pain, one might ask: do the results compare favorably with other measures of pain (for example, the judgment of an experienced observer); do the measurements yield consistently different results for conditions in which the severity of pain is generally believed to vary (e.g., minor abrasion, dental extraction, renal colic); and do the results predict pain-related behavior like sweating, moaning, or requests for medication?

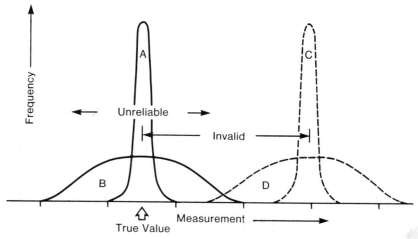

Figure 2.1.   Validity and Reliability. A is valid and reliable; B is valid but not reliable; C is not valid but is reliable; D is neither valid nor reliable.

Reliability

Reliability is the extent to which repeated measurements of a relatively stable phenomenon fall closely to each other. Repeatability, reproducibility, and precision are other words for this property.

Validity and reliability are not necessarily related to each other. It is possible to have an instrument (e.g., laboratory machine or questionnaire) which is on the average valid (accurate) but not reliable, because its results are widely scattered about the true value. On the other hand, an instrument can be very reliable, but systematically off the mark (inaccurate). These relationships are illustrated in Figure 2.1.

In clinical medicine, the validity and reliability of various measurements are accorded widely varying emphasis. On the one hand, clinical laboratories in accredited hospitals devote a great deal of attention to "quality control." For some tests as many as half of all determinations are done for calibration. Because of such stringent controls in these laboratories, the accuracy and precision (validity and reliability) of their results per se are usually not an issue, though the clinical implications of laboratory test results might be.

The quality of "bedside" observations, on the other hand, are subject to a great deal less scrutiny. This is so even though they deserve the same care as laboratory test results. The questions are the same: for example, how reproducible are our descriptions of a diastolic murmur—from doctor to doctor, and time to time; and how valid is our estimate of the degree of mitral stenosis, based on clinical findings, compared to the valve area determined at surgery? If a measurement is important, we need to consider both validity and reliability regardless of whether the measurement is made by an instrument or our own senses.

Table 2.2
Sources of Variation

Source	Definition	
Measurement		
Instrument	The means of making the measurement	
Observer	The person making the measurement	Cumulative
Biologic		
Within individuals	Changes in subjects with time and situation	
Among individuals	Biologic differences from subject to subject	

VARIATION

Clinical measurements can take on a range of values, depending on the circumstances in which they are made. Sometimes this variation can be so great that any given observation or small set of observations is likely to present a misleading representation of what it is being measured. To avoid erroneous conclusions about data, clinicians should be aware of the reasons for variation in a given situation, and which are likely to play a large part, a small part or no part at all in what has been observed.

Sources of Variation

How does variation arise? The conditions which contribute to overall variation include the act of measurement, the biologic differences within individuals from time to time, and the biologic differences from person to person (Table 2.2). The sources of variation are cumulative, so that observations subject to any one source are also subject to the ones that preceed it. This way of thinking about variation gives us a means of sorting out which sources are likely to apply in a given situation, how much they have contributed to the observed data, and how they might be reduced.

Measurement Variation

All observations are subject to variation resulting from measurement because of the performance of the instruments and observers involved in the measurement. It is possible to reduce this source of variation by making measurements with great care and following standard protocols. However, when measurements involve human judgment, rather than machines, variation can be particularly large and difficult to control. For example, when physicians specializing in tuberculosis were shown two chest X-rays taken three months apart from patients with tuberculosis and were asked to rate the second film as better, worse, or the same, their agreement with themselves on two different occasions was only 79% (2).

Variations in measurements also arise because measurements are made on a sample of the phenomenon being described. Often the "sampling fraction"—the fraction of the whole which is included in the sample—is very small. A liver biopsy represents only about 1/100,000 of the liver. Because so little of the whole is examined, there is room for considerable variation from one sample to another. If measurements are made by several different methods (e.g., different laboratories, different technicians, or different machines) some of the determinations may manifest systematic differences from the correct value, contributing to the spread of values obtained.

Biologic Variation

Variation also arises because of biologic changes within individuals over time. The true value of most biologic phenomena changes from moment to moment. A measurement at a point in time is a sample of measurements during a period of time, and may not represent the "true" value of these measurements. Yet clinical measurements are usually made at one point in time, and are assumed to apply to the subject for a period of time. The true value may thereby be misrepresented.

Example—Clinicians usually estimate the frequency of ventricular premature depolarization (VPDs) by making relatively brief observations—perhaps feeling a pulse for one minute or reviewing an electrocardiogram (as little as 10 seconds of observation). However, the frequency of VPDs in a given patient varies with time. To obtain a larger sample of VPD rate, a portable (Holter) monitor is sometimes used. But monitoring even for extended periods of time can be misleading. Figure 2.2 shows observations on one patient with VPDs, illustrative of others studied. VPDs per hour varied from less than 20 to over 380, according to day and time of day. From these data, the authors determined that "to distinguish a reduction in VPD frequency attributable to therapeutic intervention rather than biologic or spontaneous variation alone required a greater than 83%

reduction in VPD frequency if only two 24-hour monitoring periods were compared ... "(3).

Finally, variation arises because of differences among subjects. Despite all other reasons for variation, biologic differences among people predominate in many situations. For example several studies have shown that a casual blood pressure, although subject to all other forms of variation, is highly predictive of cardiovascular disease.

Sometimes important sources of variation may be discounted because it is inconvenient, even threatening, to acknowledge them. For example, when caring for a patient with ventricular arrhythmia, it would be preferable to use simple clinical observations like feeling the pulse to guide clinical decisions. Protracted monitoring is just not feasible on a

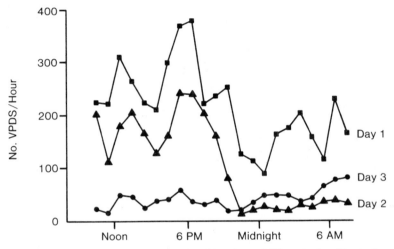

Figure 2.2. Biologic Variability. The Number of Ventricular Premature Depolarizations (VPDs) for One Untreated Patient on Three Consecutive Days. (Redrawn from Morganroth J, Michelson EJ, Horowitz LN, Josephson ME, Pearlman AS, Dunkman WB. *Circulation*, 1978; 58:408–414.)

day-to-day basis. Also, clinicians want one or another of their treatments to work, and this perfectly normal feeling may influence how they interpret the different rates they observe. As a result, the enormous variation in VPD rate within subjects may be too readily discounted. As Figure 2.2 suggests, this could be a mistake.

The several sources of variation are cumulative. Figure 2.3 illustrates this for the measurement of blood pressure. Variation due to measurement contributed relatively little, although it covered as much as a 12 mm Hg range for the various observers. On the other hand, individuals do vary a great deal from moment to moment throughout the day, so that any single blood pressure reading might be quite unrepresentative of the usual for that patient. Much of this variation is not random, because blood pressure is generally higher when awake, when excited, during visits to physicians, etc. Of course, we are most interested in the bottom curve, to know where an individual patient falls among his peers.

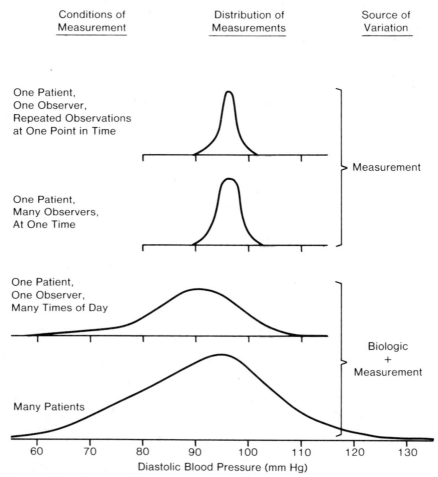

Figure 2.3.   Sources of Variation. The Measurement of Blood Pressure (Data from: Fletcher RH, and Fletcher SW. unpublished, and Boe J, Humerfelt S, Wedervang F, Oecon C. *Acta Med Scand*, 1957; 157:5–313.)

Effects of Variation

Another way of thinking about variation is in terms of its net effect on the validity of a measurement and what can be done about it.

Random variation will, on the average, result in no net misrepresentation of the true state of affairs. Inaccuracy due to random variation can be reduced by taking a larger sample of what is being measured—for example, counting more cells on a blood smear or examining a larger area of a urine sediment. Also, the extent of random variation can be estimated by means of inferential statistics (Chapter 9).

On the other hand, biased results are systematically different from the true value, no matter how many times they are repeated. For example, when investigating a patient suspected of having an infiltrative liver disease (perhaps because of an elevated serum alkaline phosphatase) a single liver biopsy may be subject to bias, depending on how the lesions are distributed in the liver. If the lesion is a metastasis in the left lobe of the liver a biopsy in the usual place (the right lobe) would be biased. On the other hand, a biopsy for miliary tuberculosis, which is represented by millions of small granulomata throughout the liver, would be inaccurate only through random variation. Similarly, all of the high values for VPD's shown in Figure 2.2 were recorded on the first day, and most of the low values on the third. The days were biased estimates of each other, because of variation in VPD rate from day-to-day.

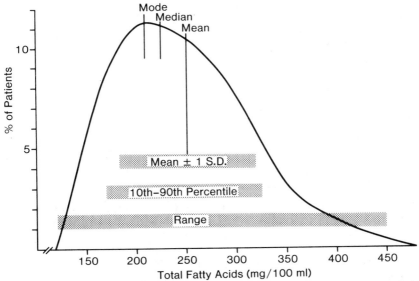

Figure 2.4. Measures of Central Tendency and Dispersion. Total Fatty Acids in Blood. (Data from: Martin HF, Gudzinowicz BJ, Fanger H. Normal Values in Clinical Chemistry, New York: Marcel Dekker, Inc., 1975.)

DISTRIBUTIONS

Data which are measured on interval scales can be presented as a table, or as a figure called a "frequency distribution" showing the number (or proportion) of a defined group of people possessing each value in the range of values in the distribution (see Figure 2.4). Presenting interval data as a figure or table conveys the information in relatively fine detail. However, it is frequently convenient to summarize distributions even further. Indeed, summarization is imperative if a large number of distributions are to be presented and compared.

Two basic properties of distributions are used to summarize them. One is *central tendency,* the middle of the distribution. The other is *dispersion,* how spread out the values are. Various ways of expressing central tendency and dispersion, along with their advantages and disadvantages, are summarized in Tables 2.3 and 2.4 and illustrated in Figure 2.4.

Table 2.3
Expressions of Central Tendency

Expression	Definition	Advantages	Disadvantages
Mean	Sum of observations / Number of observations	Well-suited for mathematical manipulation	Easily influenced by extreme values
Median	The point where the number of observations above equals the number below	Not easily influenced by extreme values	Not well-suited for mathematical manipulation
Mode	Most frequently-occuring value	Simplicity of meaning	Sometimes there are no, or many, ''most frequent'' values.

Actual Distributions

The frequency distributions of four common blood tests: potassium, glucose, alkaline phosphatase, and hemoglobin are shown in Figure 2.5. In general, most of the values appear in the middle of the distributions. The distributions are smooth, and except for the central part of the curves there are no "humps" or irregularities in the curves. The high and low ends of the distributions stretch out into tails, with the tail at one end often being more prominent than the tail at the other (i.e., the curves are "skewed" toward that end). Whereas some of the distributions are skewed toward higher values, others are skewed in the opposite direction. In other words, these distributions are unimodal and asymmetric but otherwise do not resemble each other.

The distribution of values for many laboratory tests changes with characteristics of the subjects like age, sex, race, or nutrition. Therefore, what might be a perfectly ordinary value for one person could be unusual for another. Figure 2.6 shows how the distribution of one such test, blood urea nitrogen (BUN), changes with age. A BUN of 25 mg/100 ml would be unusually high for a young person, but not particularly remarkable for an older person.

The Normal Distribution

Another kind of distribution, called the Normal or "Gaussian" distribution, should be contrasted with naturally-occurring distributions, inasmuch as the two are frequently confused. The Normal curve was first

Table 2.4
Expressions of Dispersion

Expression	Definition	Advantages	Disadvantages
Range	From lowest to highest value in a distribution	Includes all values	Greatly affected by extreme values
Standard deviation*	The absolute value of the average difference of individual values from the mean	Well-suited for mathematical manipulation	For non-Gaussian distributions, does not describe a known proportion of the observations
Percentile, decile, quartile, etc.	The proportion of all observations falling between specified values	Describes the "unusualness" of a value without assumptions about the shape of a distribution	Not well-suited for statistical manipulation

$$* \ \sqrt{\frac{\Sigma(X - \bar{X})^2}{N - 1}}$$

where: X = each observation
$\bar{X}$ = mean of all observations
N = number of observations

described by Johann Gauss, a German mathematician and physical scientist, in the 19th century. The Normal curve describes the distribution of repeated measurements of the same physical object by the same instrument. Dispersion of values represents random variation alone. A Normal curve is shown in Figure 2.7. The curve is symmetrical and bell-shaped. It also has the mathematical property that about two-thirds of the observations possess values within 1 standard deviation of the mean, and about 95% within 2 standard deviations.

Clinical distributions often resemble a Normal distribution in that they are usually smooth, unimodal, and bell-shaped. But the resemblance is

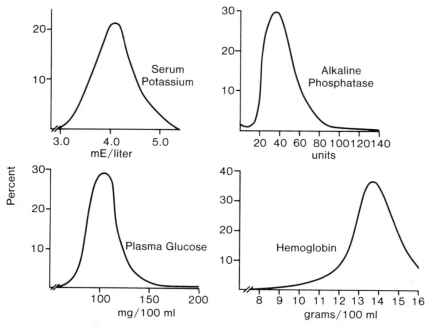

Figure 2.5. Examples of Frequency Distributions for Clinical Measurements (Data from: Martin HF, Gudzinowicz BJ, Fanger H. Normal Values in Clinical Chemistry. New York: Marcel Dekker, Inc. 1975).

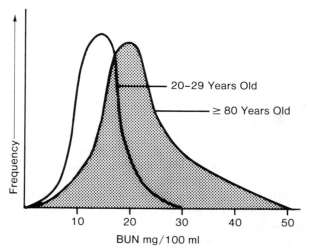

Figure 2.6. Change in Normal Function with Age. BUN in People Aged 20–29 and 80 or older. (Data from Martin HF, Gudzinowicz BJ, Fanger H. Normal Values in Clinical Chemistry. New York: Marcel Dekker, Inc., 1975.)

superficial. As one statistician put it:

> ... The experimental fact is that for most physiologic variables the distribution is smooth, unimodal, and skewed, and that mean ± 2 standard deviations does not cut off the desired 95%. We have no mathematical, statistical, or other theorems that enable us to predict the shape of the distributions of physiologic measurements (4).

Whereas the Normal distribution is derived from mathematical theory and reflects only random variation, many other sources of variation contribute to distributions of clinical measurements, particularly biologic differences among subjects. As a result, if distributions of clinical measurements from many subjects resemble Normal curves, it is largely by accident. It is important to remember this because it is often assumed, as a matter of convenience, that clinical measurements are normally distributed.

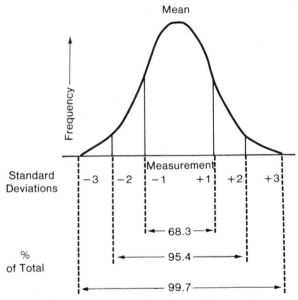

Figure 2.7. Normal (Gaussian) Distribution.

CRITERIA FOR ABNORMALITY

It would be convenient if the frequency distributions of measurements for normal and abnormal subjects were so distinct that the two populations could be recognized on a curve representing values from both populations. Figure 2.8, showing the activity of an enzyme which is inherited through a single gene, is an example of an actual distribution in which this is possible. However, usually the distributions which clinicians work with do not display sharp breaks or second peaks which distinguish normal from abnormal results.

There are several reasons why this is so. For many laboratory tests, there are not even theoretical reasons for believing that distinct populations—well and diseased—exist. Disease is acquired by degrees, and so there is a smooth transition from low to high values with increasing degrees of dysfunction. Laboratory tests reflecting organ failure, like BUN for renal failure, behave in this way. In other situations, well and diseased persons do in fact belong to separate populations. For example, the parathyroid glands of patients with hyperparathyroidism have a different histologic appearance (adenoma or hyperplasia) from normal glands, and a frequency distribution of serum calciums for the two anatomic groups would appear different. However, in unselected populations the diseased patients often do not stand out from normal people because there are very few diseased people, relative to normal people; and because laboratory values for the diseased population overlap with those for normals. The distribution curve for diseased people is "swallowed up" by the distribution curve for normal people.

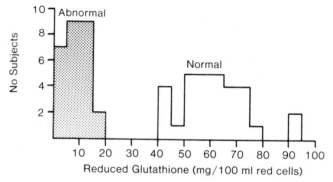

Figure 2.8. Clean Separation of Normal From Abnormal People. Assay for Reduced Glutathione in Male Relatives of Subjects with Glucose-6-Phosphate Dehydrogenase Deficiency. (Redrawn from: Childs B, Zinkham W, Browne EA, Kimbro EL, Torbert JV. *Bull Johns Hopkins Hosp*, 1958; 102:21–37.)

Example—Hyperparathyroidism is a relatively common disease, being present in approximately 1 in 200 people in the general population. Patients with confirmed hyperparathyroidism exhibit a range of serum calciums which overlaps with values commonly found in people with normal parathyroid glands, although on the average the values are higher. When serum calciums for a small number of diseased persons are part of a frequency distribution of calciums for a larger number of normal persons, the smaller population is just too small, and too much like the larger normal population, to stand out as a separate peak. Figure 2.9 illustrates these relationships.

If, on the other hand, normal and diseased populations are mixed in more equal proportions—perhaps by selecting out for testing people with an unusually high likelihood of disease—then the resulting distribution could be truly bimodal. Even so, diseased and non-diseased persons would usually not be cleanly separable (see Chapters 3 and 4).

If there is no sharp dividing line between normal and abnormal, and the clinician can choose where the line is placed, what ground rules should be used to decide?

Three criteria have proven useful: being unusual, being sick, and being treatable. For a given measurement, these approaches bear no necessary relation to each other, so that what might be considered abnormal using one criterion might be normal by another.

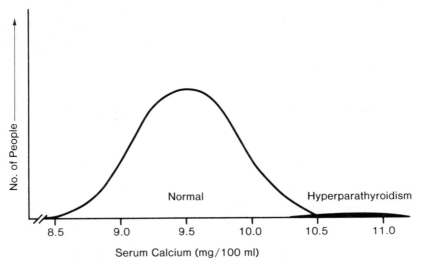

Figure 2.9. Separating Normal from Abnormal when Few of the Patients are Abnormal. Hypothetical Distribution of Serum Calciums in Normal and Hyperparathyroid People in the General Population (Prevalence of Normal/Prevalence of Hyperparathyroid 200/1).

Abnormal as Unusual

In clinical medicine, normal usually refers to the most frequently occurring or usual state of affairs. Whatever occurs often is considered normal, and what occurs infrequently is abnormal. This is a statistical definition, based on the frequency of a characteristic in a defined, usually non-diseased population. However, the reference population need not be non-diseased. We may even say it is normal to have pain after surgery.

It is tempting to be more specific, and define what is unusual in mathematical terms. One way of establishing a cut-off point between normal and abnormal is to agree, somewhat arbitrarily, that all values beyond 2 standard deviations from the mean are abnormal. On the assumption that the distribution in question approximates a normal or Guassian distribution, 2.5% of observations would then appear in each tail of a distribution, and be considered abnormal.

Of course, as already pointed out, most biologic measurements are not normally distributed. So it has been suggested that unusual values, whatever the proportion chosen, are better expressed as percentiles of the underlying distribution. In this way, it is possible to make a direct statement about how infrequent a value is, without making assumptions about the shape of the distribution from which it came.

This statistical definition of normality serves adequately in some situations. But there are several ways in which it can be ambiguous or misleading.

1. If all values beyond an arbitrary statistical limit—for example, the 95th percentile—were considered abnormal, then the prevalence of all diseases, would be the same, 5%. But in our usual way of thinking about disease frequency, prevalence varies a great deal.

2. There is no general relationship between the degree of statistical unusualness and clinical disease. The relationship is specific to the disease in question. For some measurements, deviations from usual are associated with disease to an important degree only at quite extreme values, well beyond the 95th or even the 99th percentile.

Example—The World Health Organization considers anemia to be present when hemoglobin (Hb) levels are below 12 grams/100 ml in adult non-pregnant females. In a British survey of women age 20–64, Hb for 11% of 920 non-pregnant women fell below 12 grams. But were they "diseased" in any way, by virtue of their low Hb? Two possibilities come to mind: the low Hb may be associated with symptoms; or it may be a marker for serious underlying disease. Symptoms like fatigue, dizziness, and irritability were not correlated with Hb level, at least for women whose Hb was above 8.0. Moreover, oral iron, given to women with Hb between 8.0 and 12.0, increased their Hb by an average of 2.30 grams/100 ml but did not lead to any greater improvement in symptoms than was experienced by women given placebo. As for serious underlying disease, it is true that occasionally low Hb may be a manifestation of cancer, chronic infection or rheumatic conditions. But only a very small proportion of women with low Hb have these conditions.

Thus, only at Hb levels below 8.0, which occurred in less than 1% of these women, might anemia be an important health problem (5).

3. Some extreme values are distinctly unsual, but preferable to more usual ones. This is particularly true at the low end of some distributions. Who would not be pleased to have a serum creatinine of 0.3 mg/100 ml or a systolic blood pressure of 100 mm Hg.? Both are unusually low, but they represent better than average health or risk.

4. Sometimes patients are clearly diseased, even though laboratory tests diagnostic of their disease are in the usual range for healthy people. Examples include low pressure hydrocephalus, normal pressure glaucoma and normocalcemic hyperparathyroidism.

5. Many laboratory tests are related to risk of disease over their entire

range of values, from low to high. Figure 2.10 illustrates how one such test, serum cholesterol, is related to coronary heart disease. There is an almost 3-fold increase in risk from the "low normal" to the "high normal" range.

It is possible that changes for individuals, occurring within the normal range, could have physiologic significance. As an example, consider changes in serum levels of thyroxine (T_4). The normal limits for serum T_4 are taken to be 5.0–11.0 mg/100 ml. Suppose an individual's T_4 is usually around 10.9. If that person were to experience a fall in T_4 to 5.1, unassociated with a change in serum proteins or the proportion of T_4 bound, the lower value would also fall within the range of normal. Would the lower value be physiologic for that patient? In fact, such falls in T_4

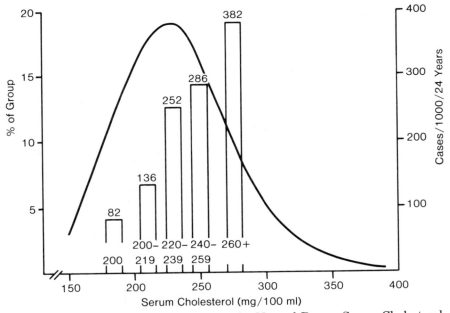

Figure 2.10. Increasing Risk Through the Normal Range. Serum Cholesterol and the Risk of Coronary Heart Disease in Men Aged 30–39. (Adapted from: Dawber TR, The Framingham Study. Cambridge: Harvard U. Press, 1980.)

have been associated with elevations in thyroid-stimulating hormone, suggesting that the lower level has been recognized by the pituitary as too low.

Abnormal as Associated with Disease

A sounder approach to distinguishing normal from abnormal is to call abnormal those observations that are regularly associated with disease, disability, or death, where disease means any clinically meaningful departure from good health, whether it be manifested directly by symptoms, or indirectly by observations which are themselves strongly associated with poor health (e.g., "risk factors" or clinically important physical signs). This caveat is mentioned in order to avoid the kind of circular reasoning whereby statistically-unusual measurements are called diseases, and the unusualness is found to be a good predictor of disease.

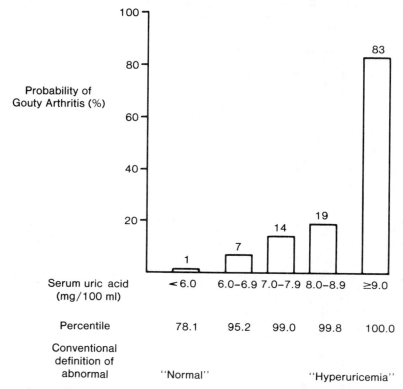

Figure 2.11.   The Relationship between Normal and the Risk of Disease. The Risk for Men of Having Gouty Arthritis at Various Levels of Serum Uric Acid. (Data from: Hall AP, Barry PE, Dawber TR, McNamara P. *Am J Med*, 1967; 42:27–37.)

Judgments about what is an important risk may vary, even where the risk is known (Figure 2.11). Most would agree that the risk of developing gout is negligible at uric acid levels below 7.0 mg/100 ml (this includes 95.2% of the population). After that, the risk starts to rise so that at levels greater than 9.0, nearly everyone will develop gout. The decision as to where abnormal lies is a matter of judgment about the level of risk worth preventing, given current methods. It is conventional to choose that value around 8.0 or 9.0 mg/100 ml.

Abnormal as Treatable

For some conditions, particularly those which are not troublesome in their own right (i.e., are asymptomatic), it is better to consider a measurement abnormal if its treatment leads to a better outcome. This is because not everything that marks risk can be successfully treated. Removal of risk factors may not remove risk, either because the factor is not itself a cause of disease, but only related to a cause, or because irreversible damage has already occurred.

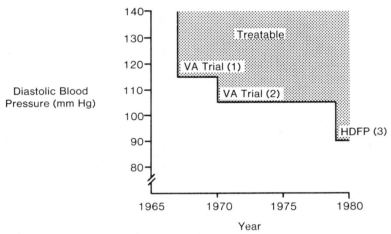

Figure 2.12.   The Changing Definition of Treatable Disease. Accumulating Evidence for Treating Successively Lower Levels of Blood Pressure. (Data from: 1. Veterans Administration Cooperative Study Group on Antihypertensive Agents. *JAMA*, 1967; 202:1028–1034. 2. Veterans Administration Cooperative Study Group on Hypertensive Agents. *JAMA*, 1970; 213:1143–1152. 3. Hypertension Detection and Follow-up Program (HDFP) Cooperative Group. *JAMA*, 1979; 242:2562–2570.)

What we consider treatable changes with time. At their best, therapeutic decisions are grounded on evidence in the form of well-conducted clinical trials (Chapter 8). As new knowledge accumulates from the results of clinical trials, the level at which treatment is believed valuable may change. Figure 2.12 shows how accumulating evidence for treating hypertension has changed our definition of what level is treatable. With the passage of time, successively lower levels of diastolic blood pressure have been shown to be worth treating.

REGRESSION TO THE MEAN

When clinicians encounter an unexpectedly abnormal test result, they tend to repeat it. Often the second test result is closer to normal and they are reassured. Why does this happen?

Patients selected because they represent an extreme value in a distribution can be expected, on the average, to have less extreme values on subsequent measurements. This can occur for purely statistical reasons (random variation) and is called *regression to the mean.*

Example—In a trial of the effect of reducing multiple risk factors on the subsequent incidence of coronary heart disease, (The Multiple Risk Factor Intervention Trial), high risk patients were selected for study. Elevated blood pressure was one of the risk factors that caused people to be considered for the study. Subjects were screened for inclusion in the study on three consecutive visits. Table 2.5 shows blood pressures at those visits, before any therapeutic interventions were undertaken.

There was a substantial fall in mean blood pressure between the first and the third visit. The authors attributed this fall to regression to the mean, as well as a tendency for patients to be more relaxed on later visits. (There was also a fall in serum cholesterol, which presumably was not affected by moment-to-moment anxiety) (6).

Table 2.5

An Example of Regression to the Mean. Diastolic Blood Pressure for Patients Selected because of a High Value on Three Consecutive Visits.*

Visit	Diastolic Blood Pressure (mm Hg)	
	Mean	S.D.
1	99.2	7.7
2	91.2	9.6
3	90.7	9.8

* Data from: Kuller L, Neaton J, Cagginall A, Falvao-Gerard L. *Am J Epid,* 1980; 112:185–199.

Regression to the mean arose in the following way. Subjects were first selected because their initial blood pressure fell above an arbitrarily selected cut-off point in the tail of a distribution of blood pressures for all the patients examined. Some of those subjects would consistently fall above the cut-off point on subsequent measurements as well, because their true blood pressures were ordinarily higher than average. But others who were found to have blood pressures above the cut-off point during the initial screening usually had lower pressure readings. They were included only because they happened, through random variation, to have high blood pressures at that point in time. When people whose measurements were above the cut-off point at the first visit were re-examined those with usually lower blood pressures had, on the average, lower values than on the first visit. This tended to drag downward the mean blood pressure of the subgroup originally found to have readings above the cut-point.

Thus, patients who are singled out from others because they possess a laboratory test which is unusually high can be expected, on the average, to be closer to normal if the test is repeated. What is more, subsequent values are likely to be more accurate estimates of the true value, which could be obtained if the measurement were repeated for a particular patient many times. So the time-honored practice of repeating laboratory tests which are found to be abnormal and calling the second one, which is often within normal limits, the correct one is not just wishful thinking. It has a sound theoretical basis. It also has an empirical basis. For example, it has been shown that half of serum T_4 tests found to be outside normal limits on screening were within normal limits when repeated (7). However, the more extreme the initial reading is, the less likely it is to be normal if it is repeated.

SUMMARY

Clinical observations are measured on nominal, ordinal, or interval scales. They are found to vary because of measurement error, differences in individuals from time to time, and differences among individuals.

Clinicians often find it useful to simplify data, by calling them normal or abnormal, in order to communicate more efficiently or select a course of action. However, there is usually no inherent dividing line between normal and abnormal. The shapes of frequency distributions for clinical observations follow no general rules. Abnormal subjects are often not conceptually distinct from normal subjects, and they possess values which overlap with those for normals.

The choice of a point at which normal becomes abnormal is based on data about the consequences of possessing a given value for the measurement in question—for example, of being statistically unusual, being associated with disease, or being treatable. In any case, if extreme values in a distribution are singled out for special attention, they are likely to fall closer to the usual if they are repeated, for purely statistical reasons called regression to the mean.

Suggested Reading

Feinstein AR. Clinical Judgement. Baltimore: Williams & Wilkins Co., 1967.

Wulff HR. Rational Diagnosis and Treatment. Oxford: Blackwell Scientific Publications, 1976.

Galen RS, Gambino SR. Beyond Normality. New York: John Wiley & Sons, 1975.

Feinstein AR. Section 3. Problems in measurement. Clinical Biostatistics, St. Louis, C.V. Mosby Co., 1977.

Martin HF, Gudzinowicz BJ, Fanger H. Normal Values in Clinical Chemistry. New York: Marcel Dekker, Inc. 1975.

Koran LM. The reliability of clinical methods, data and judgment. N Engl J Med, 1975; 293:642–646, 695–701.

Mainland D. Remarks on clinical "norms". Clin Chem, 1971; 17:267–274.

References

1. Feinstein AR. The need for humanized science in evaluating medication. Lancet, 1972; 2:421–423.
2. Koran L. The reliability of clinical methods, data and judgment. N Engl J Med, 1975; 293:642–646, 695–701.
3. Morganroth J, Michelson EL, Horowitz LN, Josephson ME, Pearlman AS, Dunkman

WB. Limitations of routine long-term electrocardiographic monitoring to assess ventricular ectopic frequency. *Circulation*, 1978; 58:408–414.

4. Elveback LR, Guillier CL, Keating FR. Health normality, and the ghost of Gauss. *JAMA*, 1970; 211:69–75.

5. Elwood PC, Waters WE, Greene WTW, Sweetnam P. Symptoms and circulating hemoglobin level. *J Chron Dis*, 1969; 21:615–628.

6. Kuller L, Neaton J, Caggiula A, Falvao-Gerard L. Primary prevention of heart attacks: the multiple risk factor intervention trial. *Am J Epid* 1980; 112:185–199.

7. Epstein KA, Schneiderman LJ, Bush JW, Zettner A. The "abnormal" screening serum thyroxine (T_4): analysis of physician response, outcome, cost and health effectiveness. *J Chron Dis*, 1981; 34:175–190.

chapter

3

Diagnostic Test

Clinicians devote a great deal of time to determining diagnoses for complaints or abnormalities presented by their patients, arriving at the diagnoses after applying various diagnostic tests. Even so, few practicing physicians receive formal training in the interpretation of diagnostic tests. Most competent clinicians use good judgment, a thorough knowledge of the literature, and a kind of rough and ready approach to how the information should be organized. However, there are also basic principles with which a clinician should be familiar when interpreting diagnostic tests. This chapter will deal with those principles.

A "diagnostic test" ordinarily is taken to mean a test performed in a laboratory. But the principles to be discussed in this chapter apply equally well to clinical information obtained from history, physical examination, or X-rays. They also apply where a constellation of findings serves as a diagnostic test. Thus, one might speak of the value of arthritis, carditis, and chorea in diagnosing rheumatic fever or of hemoptysis and weight loss in a cigarette smoker as an indicator of lung cancer.

SIMPLIFYING DATA

In the previous chapter, it was pointed out that clinical measurements (including data from diagnostic tests) are expressed on nominal, ordinal, or interval scales. Regardless of the kind of data produced by diagnostic tests, clinicians are inclined to reduce the data to a simpler form in order to make it useful in practice. Most ordinal scales are examples of this simplification process. Obviously, heart murmurs can vary from very loud to inaudible. But expressing subtle gradations in the intensity of murmurs is both tedious and unnecessary. A simple ordinal scale, grade I to VI, serves just as well (Figure 3.1). More often, complex data are reduced to a simple dichotomy—for example, present/absent, abnormal/normal, or diseased/well. This is particularly so when test results are used to decide on treatment. At any given point in time, therapeutic decisions are either/or decisions. Either treatment is begun or it is withheld.

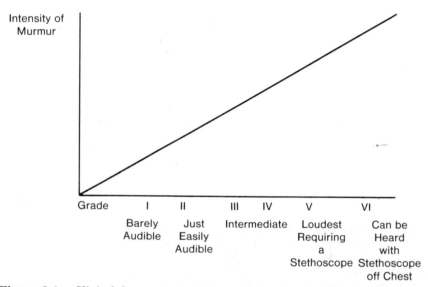

Figure 3.1. Clinical Conversion of Interval Data to an Ordinal Scale: Grading the Intensity of Heart Murmurs. Note that the Distances between the Grades are not Necessarily of Equal Size.

The use of blood pressure data to decide on therapy is an example of how we simplify information for practical purposes. Blood pressure is ordinarily measured to the nearest millimeter of mercury—that is, on an interval scale. However, most physicians choose a particular level (e.g., 90 mm Hg diastolic pressure) at which they initiate treatment. In doing so, they have transformed interval into nominal (in this case, dichotomous) data. To take the example further, it may be that a physician would choose a treatment plan according to whether the patient's diastolic blood pressure is "mildly elevated" (90–104 mm Hg), "moderately elevated" (105–114 mm Hg) or "severely elevated" (115 mm Hg and above). The doctor would then be reacting to the test in an ordinal manner.

THE ACCURACY OF A TEST RESULT

As all clinicians quickly learn, establishing diagnoses is an imperfect process, resulting in a probability rather than a certainty of being right. That being the case, it behooves the clinician to become famililar with the mathematical relationships between the properties of diagnostic tests and the information they yield in various clinical situations. In many instances, understanding these issues will help the clinician resolve some uncertainty surrounding the use of diagnostic tests. In other situations, it may only increase understanding of the uncertainty. Occasionally, it may convince the clinician to increase his uncertainty!

		Disease: Present	Disease: Absent
Test	Positive	True Positive	False Positive
	Negative	False Negative	True Negative

Figure 3.2. The Relationship between a Diagnostic Test Result and the Occurrence of Disease. There are Two Possibilities for the Result to be Correct (True Positive and True Negative) and Two Possibilities for the Result to be Incorrect (False Positive and False Negative).

A simple way of looking at the relationships between a test's results and the true diagnosis is shown in Figure 3.2. The test is considered to be either positive (abnormal) or negative (normal) and the disease either present or absent. There are then four possible interpretations of test results, two of which are correct, and two wrong. The test has given the correct answer when it is positive in the presence of disease, or negative in the absence of the disease. On the other hand, the test has been misleading if it is positive when the disease is absent (false positive), or negative when the disease is present (false negative).

The "Gold Standard"

Assessment of the test's accuracy rests on its relationship to some way of knowing whether the disease is truly present or not—a sound assessment of the truth. As it turns out, this gold standard is often elusive. Sometimes the standard of accuracy is itself a relatively simple and inexpensive test, like a throat culture for Group A β-hemolytic strepto-coccus to validate the clinical impression of strep throat. However, this is usually not the case. More often, one must turn to relatively elaborate, expensive, or risky tests in order to be certain whether the disease is present or absent. Among these are tissue diagnoses, radiologic contrast procedures, prolonged follow-up—and, of course, autopsies.

Because it is almost always more costly, and sometimes less feasible, to use these more accurate ways of establishing the truth, simpler tests are often substituted for the rigorous gold standard, at least initially. Chest X-rays and sputum smears are used to determine the nature of pneumonia rather than lung biopsy with examination of the diseased lung tissue. Similarly, electrocardiograms and serum enzymes are ordinarily used to establish the diagnosis of acute myocardial infarction, rather than biopsy. The simpler tests are used as proxies for more elaborate but more accurate ways of establishing the presence of disease with the understand-ing that some risk of misclassification results, which is justified by the feasibility of the simpler tests.

It would be helpful if our commonly used diagnostic tests were all backed by sound data comparing their accuracy to an appropriate stan-dard. The goal of all clinical studies describing the value of diagnostic tests should be to obtain data for all four of the cells in Figure 3.2. Without all these data, it is not possible to answer important questions about the performance of the tests.

Lack of Information on Negative Tests

Given that the goal is to fill in all of the four cells, it must be stated that sometimes this is difficult to do in the real world. It may be that an objective and valid means of establishing the diagnosis exists, but is not available for the purposes of formally establishing the properties of a diagnostic test for ethical or practical reasons. Consider the situation in which most information about diagnostic tests is obtained. Published accounts come primarily from clinical, and not research, settings. Under these circumstances, physicians are using the test in the process of caring for patients. They ordinarily feel justified in proceeding with more exhaustive evaluation, in the patient's best interest, only when prelimi-nary diagnostic tests are positive. They are naturally reluctant to initiate an aggressive work-up, with its associated risk and expense, when the test is negative. As a result, information on negative tests, whether true negative or false negative, tends to be much less complete in the medical literature.

This problem is illustrated by a recent study of the relative merits of two tests for diagnosing gallstones—a new diagnostic test, ultrasonic cholecystography, and the conventional test, radiographic cholecystog-raphy (1). If patients had abnormal radiographic cholecystograms, they were submitted to surgery where the true diagnosis of gallstones could be confirmed or rejected. However, patients with normal oral cholecysto-grams were not sent to surgery, whether or not ultrasound indicated stones. The authors understandably considered it unethical by current medical standards to submit patients to surgery on the basis of a new and unproven test. Nevertheless, the situation leaves us unable to determine the false negative rate for oral cholecystograms, or for any of the ultrasound results that were accompanied by a negative oral cholecystogram.

For diseases which are not self-limited, and ordinarily become overt in a matter of a few years after they are first suspected, the results of follow-up can serve as a gold standard. Most cancers and chronic, degenerative diseases fall into this category. For them, validation is possible even if on-the-spot confirmation of a test's performance is not feasible because the immediately-available gold standard is too risky, involved, or expensive. All it takes is time and patience.

Lack of Objective Standards for Disease

For some conditions, there are simply no hard and fast criteria for diagnosis. Angina pectoris is one of these. The clinical manifestations were described nearly a century ago, and are familiar to all medical students and many laymen as well. Yet there is still no better way to substantiate the presence of angina pectoris than a carefully taken history. Certainly a great many objectively measurable phenomena are related to this clinical syndrome—for example, the presence of coronary lesions seen on angiography, increased concentrations of lactate in coronary sinus blood, and characteristic abnormalities on electrocardiograms both at rest and with exercise. All are more commonly found in patients believed to have angina pectoris. But none is so uniquely tied to the clinical syndrome that it will serve as the standard by which the condition is considered present or absent.

Sometimes, usually in an effort to be "rigorous", circular reasoning is applied. The validity of a laboratory test is established by comparing its results to a clinical diagnosis, based on a careful history of symptoms and a physical examination. Once established, the test is then used to validate the clinical diagnosis gained from history and physical examination! An example would be the use of manometry to "confirm" irritable bowel syndrome, because the contraction pattern demonstrated by manometry and believed characteristic of irritable bowel was validated by clinical impression in the first place.

Consequences of Imperfect Standards

Because of difficulties like these, it is frequently not possible for physicians in practice to find information on how well the tests they use compare to a thoroughly trustworthy standard. They must choose as their standard of validity another test which admittedly is imperfect but is considered the best available. This may force them into comparing one weak test against another, one being taken as a standard of validity because it has had longer use or is considered superior by a consensus of experts. In doing so, a paradox may arise. If a new test is compared with an old (but inaccurate) standard test, the new test may seem worse even when it is actually better. For example, if the new test is more sensitive than the standard test, the additional patients identified by the new test would be considered false positives in relation to the old test. Just such a situation occurred in a comparison of real time ultrasonography and oral cholecystography for the detection of gallstones (2). In five patients, ultrasound was positive for stones that were missed on adequate chole-cystogram. Two of the patients later underwent surgery and gallstones were found, so that for at least those two patients, the standard oral cholecystogram was actually less accurate than the new real time ultra-sound. Similarly, if the new test is more often negative in patients who really do not have the disease, results for those patients will be considered false negatives compared to the old test. Thus, if an inaccurate standard of validity is used, a new test can perform no better than that standard and will seem inferior when it approximates the truth more closely.

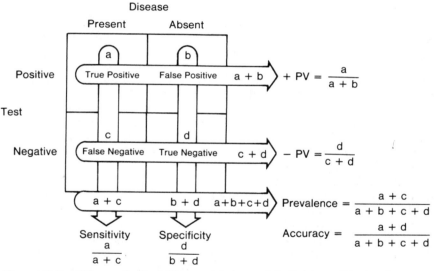

Figure 3.3.   Diagnostic Test Characteristics and Definitions. (Design Courtesy of the Department of Clinical Epidemiology and Biostatistics, McMaster Health Sciences Centre).

SENSITIVITY AND SPECIFICITY

Figure 3.3 summarizes some relationships between a diagnostic test and the actual presence of disease. It is an expansion of Figure 3.2, with the addition of some useful definitions. Most of the rest of this chapter will deal with these relationships in detail. Figure 3.4 illustrates the relationships. The diagnostic test is housestaff's clinical impression of whether patients' complaining of pharyngitis have a Group A β-hemolytic streptococcus infection or not. The gold standard is a throat culture.

Definitions

As can be seen in Figure 3.3, *sensitivity* is defined as the proportion of subjects with the disease who have a positive test for the disease. A sensitive test will rarely miss people with the disease. *Specificity* is the proportion of subjects without the disease who have a negative test. A specific test will rarely misclassify people without the disease as diseased.

Applying these definitions to the pharyngitis example, 37 of the 149 patients with sore throats had positive cultures and housestaff correctly diagnosed 27 of these—for a sensitivity of 73%. On the other hand, 112 patients had negative culture results; housestaff correctly withheld antibiotics from 77, for a specificity of 69%.

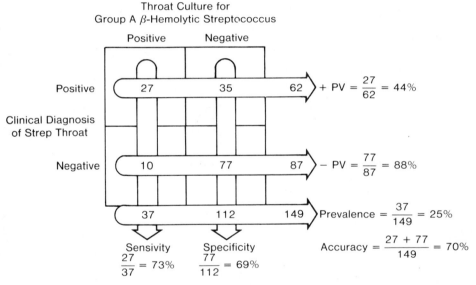

Figure 3.4. Comparison of Clinical Diagnosis with Throat Culture Results for Streptococcal Pharyngitis. (Data from: Fletcher SW, Hamann C. *J Comm Health*, 1976; 1:196–204.)

Uses of Sensitive Tests

Clinicians should take sensitivity and specificity of a diagnostic test into account when a test is selected. A sensitive test, i.e., one that is usually positive in the presence of disease, should be chosen when there is an important penalty for missing a disease. This would be so, for example, when there is reason to suspect a dangerous but treatable condition such as tuberculosis, syphilis or Hodgkin's Disease. Sensitive tests are also helpful during the early stages of a diagnostic work-up, when a great many possibilities are being considered, in order to reduce the number of possibilities. Diagnostic tests are being used in these situations to "rule out" diseases—that is, establish that certain diseases are unlikely possibilities. For example, one might choose a tuberculin skin test early in the evaluation of lung infiltrates because this test is usually positive in people with active tuberculosis. Finally, sensitive tests are useful when the probability of disease is relatively low, and the purpose of the test is to discover disease. This is the case when the test is used to screen people without complaints, as in the periodic health examination (discussed in Chapter 4). In sum, a sensitive test is most helpful to the clinician when the test result is negative.

Uses of Specific Tests

Specific tests are useful to confirm (or "rule in") a diagnosis that has been suggested by other data. This is because a highly specific test is rarely positive in the absence of disease—that is, it gives few false positive results. Highly specific tests are particularly needed when false positive

Table 3.1

Trade-Off between Sensitivity and Specificity when Diagnosing Diabetes*

Blood Sugar Level 2 Hours after Eating (mg/100 ml)	Sensitivity (%)	Specificity (%)
70	98.6	8.8
80	97.1	25.5
90	94.3	47.6
100	88.6	69.8
110	85.7	84.1
120	71.4	92.5
130	64.3	96.9
140	57.1	99.4
150	50.0	99.6
160	47.1	99.8
170	42.9	100.0
180	38.6	100.0
190	34.3	100.0
200	27.1	100.0

* From: Diabetes Program Guide, Public Health Service Publication No. 506, 1960.

results can harm the patient physically, emotionally, or financially. Thus, before patients are subjected to cancer chemotherapy, with all its attendant risks, emotional trauma, and financial costs, tissue diagnosis is generally required instead of relying upon less specific tests. In sum, a specific test is most helpful when the test result is positive.

Trade-offs between Sensitivity and Specificity

Generally there is a trade-off between the sensitivity and specificity of a diagnostic test. It is obviously desirable to have a test which is both highly sensitive and highly specific. Unfortunately, this is frequently not possible.

A trade-off between sensitivity and specificity is required when clinical data take on a range of values. In those situations, the location of a cut-off point between normal and abnormal is an arbitrary decision. As a consequence, for any given test result expressed on an interval scale, one characteristic (e.g., sensitivity) can only be increased at the expense of the other (e.g., specificity). Table 3.1 demonstrates this interrelationship for the diagnosis of diabetes. If we require that a blood sugar two hours after eating be greater than 180 mg% to diagnose diabetes, all of the people diagnosed as "diabetic" would certainly have the disease, but many other people with diabetes would be missed using this extremely demanding definition of the disease. The test would be very specific at

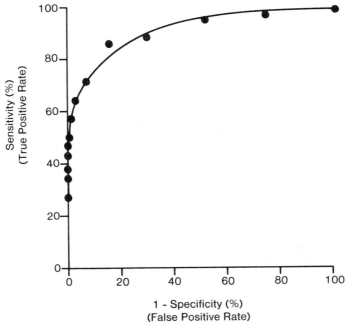

Figure 3.5. Receiver Operator Characteristic Curve of Blood Sugar Determinations in Diagnosing Diabetes.

the expense of sensitivity. At the other extreme, if anyone with a blood sugar of greater than 70 mg% were diagnosed as diabetic, very few people with the disease would be missed, but most normal people would be falsely labelled as having diabetes. The test would then be very sensitive but non-specific.

Another way to express this relationship is to construct a figure plotting the true positive rate (sensitivity) against the false positive rate (1-specificity). This relationship is called the *Receiver Operator Character-istic* of the test (ROC), and is illustrated in Figure 3.5. A ROC curve visually demonstrates the trade-off between sensitivity and specificity for a single test, in this case blood sugar. There is no way, using a single blood sugar determination under standard conditions, that one can improve both the sensitivity and specificity of the test at the same time.

Whenever a test is sensitive but not specific there is a penalty to pay. Using a highly sensitive test requires that a large number of patients with false positive results be evaluated. For example, a tuberculin test to investigate patients with lung infiltrates will produce many people with positive tests because of past exposure, or infection with atypical myco-

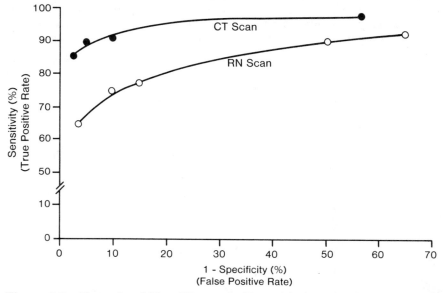

Figure 3.6. Example of New Diagnostic Test with Superior Sensitivity and Specificity Compared to an Older Test: Receiver Operator Characteristic Curves for Computerized Tomography (*CT*) and Radionuclide Scanning (*RN*) in Diagnosing Brain Tumors. (Redrawn from: Griner PF, Mayewski RJ, Mushlin AI, Greenland P. *Ann Intern Med*, 1981; 94:553–600.)

bacteria, but in whom further evaluation will determine that the infiltrates are not caused by tuberculosis. In these patients, the tuberculin test has been misleading. However, in the case of serious and treatable disease, the clinician may be willing to accept the price of misleading preliminary information in some patients.

Although clinicians are forced to make a trade-off between sensitivity and specificity for any given test, it is possible that a new test can be both more sensitive and more specific than its predecessors. The fluorescent treponemal antibody absorption test (FTA-ABS) for syphilis is both more sensitive and more specific than older tests, like those for anticardiolipin antibody (e.g., VDRL). Similarly, Figure 3.6 compares the ROC curves for two tests used to diagnose brain tumors—computerized tomography and radionuclide scanning. Computerized tomography is both more sensitive and more specific than the older "brain scan."

Obviously, tests which are both sensitive and specific are highly sought after, and can be of enormous value. However, practicing clinicians rarely work with tests which are both highly sensitive and specific. So for the present, we must use other means for getting around the trade-off between sensitivity and specificity. The most common way is to use the results of several tests together (see Chapter 4).

ESTABLISHING SENSITIVITY AND SPECIFICITY

Not infrequently, a new diagnostic test is described in glowing terms when first introduced, only to be found wanting later, when more experience with it has accumulated. Enthusiasm for the clinical value of carcinoembryonic antigen (CEA) waxed and then waned in this way. At first, CEA was considered a very promising means of diagnosing colon cancer. But CEA, subsequently, was shown to be present in a wide variety of other malignancies, as well as in approximately 20% of smokers without cancer. This kind of confusion—initial enthusiasm followed by disappointment—arises not from any dishonesty on the part of early investigators or unfair skepticism by the medical community. Rather, it is related to misunderstandings—by the investigators, the readers, or both—about how the properties of diagnostic tests are established.

At the crudest level, the properties of a diagnostic test may be inaccurately described because an improper standard of validity has been chosen, as discussed previously. However, two other issues related to the selection of diseased and non-diseased patients can profoundly affect the determination of sensitivity and specificity as well. They are the spectrum of patients to which the test is applied, and bias in judging the test's performance.

The Spectrum of Patients

Difficulties may arise when patients used to describe the test's properties are different from those to whom the test will be applied in clinical practice. Early reports of a test often assess its value among persons who are clearly diseased as compared to persons who are clearly not diseased. The test may be able to distinguish between these extremes very well. But, except in screening situations, there is no need for such a diagnostic test, because the differences between diseased and well subjects are usually obvious even without the test. What is usually needed by the clinician is a test that will distinguish between one disease and another among patients with similar symptoms, all of whom are suspected of having a particular disease.

Often tests which are very sensitive and specific in distinguishing diseased from well people are considerably less useful in distinguishing people with a given disease from people with other diseases, when both groups have similar complaints.

Example—Vacuolization of neutrophils has been suggested as a useful test for the rapid diagnosis of bacteremia, before blood culture results are available. It was noted that vacuolization occurs with considerable regularity in patients with bacteremia, and infrequently in a variety of patients without bacteremia.

However, it has not been established that the test can distinguish between patients with and without bacteremia, taken from a group in which sepsis is suspected. The test may be less effective if patients with other stressful conditions—e.g. hypovolemic shock or severe viral infections—also have vacuolization of their neutrophils and, therefore, may not be particularly useful in the clinical situation in which it might be most needed. In fact, specificity was 86% when diseased febrile bacteremic patients were compared to controls without fever or suspected sepsis, but fell to 67% when the controls were febrile, with bacterial infection but negative blood cultures. (3)

This test, therefore, is not particularly helpful in the clinical situation in which it might be used. It is not, after all, necessary to develop special means to distinguish patients suspected of having sepsis from healthy people. Simple bedside observations will suffice for that!

Bias

Sometimes the sensitivity and specificity of a test is not established independently of the means by which the true diagnosis is established, leading to a biased assessment of its properties. This may occur in several ways.

As already pointed out, if the test is evaluated using data obtained during the course of a clinical evaluation of patients suspected of having the disease in question, a positive test may prompt the clinician to continue pursuing the diagnosis, increasing the likelihood that the disease will be found. On the other hand, a negative test may cause the clinician to abandon further testing, making it more likely that the disease, if present, will be missed. In other situations, the test result may be part of the information used to establish the diagnosis; or, conversely, the results of the test may be interpreted taking other clinical information or the final diagnosis into account.

Radiologists are frequently subject to this kind of bias when they read X-rays. Because X-ray interpretation is somewhat subjective, it is easy to be influenced by the clinical information provided. All clinicians experience the situation of having X-rays over-read because of a clinical impression, or conversely, going back over old X-rays in which a finding was missed because a clinical event was not known at the time and, therefore, attention was not directed to the particular area in the X-ray. Because of these biases, some radiologists prefer to read X-rays twice, first without, and then with, the clinical information.

All of these biases tend to increase the agreement between the test and the standard of validity. That is, they tend to make the test seem more useful than it actually is.

PREDICTIVE VALUE

As noted previously, sensitivity and specificity are properties of a test which are taken into account when a decision is made whether or not to order the test. But once the results of a diagnostic test are available, whether positive or negative, the sensitivity and specificity of the test are no longer of primary importance. This is because these values give the probability that a test will be positive or negative in persons known to have or not to have the disease. But if one knew the disease status of the patient, it would not be necessary to order the test! For the clinician, the dilemma is to determine whether or not the patient has the disease, given the results of a test.

Definitions

The probability of disease, given the results of a test, is called the *predictive value* of the test (Figure 3.3). Positive predictive value is the probability of disease in a patient with a positive (abnormal) test result. Negative predictive value is the probability of *not* having the disease when the test result is negative (normal). Predictive value is an answer to the question: If my patient's test result is positive (negative), what are the chances that my patient does (does not) have the disease? Figure 3.4 illustrates these concepts. Among the patients treated with antibiotics for streptococcal pharyngitis, less than one-half (44%) had the condition by culture (positive predictive value). The negative predictive value of the housestaff's diagnostic impressions was better; of the 87 patients thought not to have streptococcal pharyngitis, the impression was correct for 77 (88%).

Terms summarizing the overall value of a test have been described. One such term, *accuracy*, is the proportion of all test results, both positive and negative, which are correct. (For the pharyngitis example in Figure 3.4, the accuracy of housestaff's diagnostic impressions was 70%.) In most cases, however, this summary term is too crude to be useful clinically because specific information about the component parts—which is what doctors need—is lost when they are aggregated into a single index.

Determinants of Predictive Value

The predictive value of a test is not a property of the test alone. It is determined by the sensitivity and specificity of the test and the prevalence of disease in the population being tested,* where prevalence has its customary meaning: the proportion of persons in a defined population at a given point in time with the condition in question. (For a full discussion of prevalence, see Chapter 5.)

As evident in Figure 3.3, the more sensitive a test is, the better will be

---

* The mathematical formula relating positive predictive value to sensitivity, specificity and prevalence is calculated according to Bayes' theorem of conditional probability:

$$+ PV = \frac{(Se)\ (P)}{(Se)\ (P) + (1\text{-}Sp)\ (1\text{-}P)}$$

where: Se = sensitivity;
       Sp = specificity;
        P = prevalence.
    +PV = positive predictive value.

the negative predictive value of the test (the more confident the clinician can be that a patient with a negative test result does not have the disease being sought). Conversely, the more specific the test is, the better will be the positive predictive value of the test.

Because predictive value is also influenced by prevalence, it is not independent of the setting in which the test is used. Positive results even for a very specific test, when applied to patients with a low likelihood of having the disease, will be largely false positives. Similarly, negative results, even for a very sensitive test, when applied to patients with a high chance of having the disease, are likely to be false negatives. In sum, the interpretation of a positive or negative diagnostic test result should vary from setting to setting, according to estimated prevalence of disease in the particular setting.

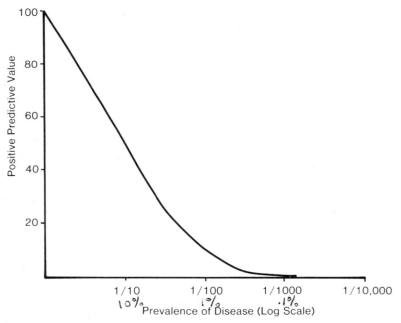

Figure 3.7. The Relationship Between Prevalence and Positive Predictive Value. (Where Sensitivity = 90% and Specificity = 90%.)

This principle is not intuitively obvious to many physicians. For them, it might help to consider how a test would perform at the extremes of prevalence. Remember that no matter how sensitive and specific a test might be (short of perfection), there will still be a small proportion of patients that are misclassified by it. Imagine a population in which no one has the disease. In such a group all positive results, even for a very specific test, will be false positives. Therefore, as the prevalence of disease in a population approaches zero, the positive predictive value of a test also approaches zero. Conversely, if everyone in a population tested has the disease, all negative results will be false negatives, even for a very sensitive test. As prevalence approaches 100%, negative predictive value approaches zero. Another way for the skeptic to convince himself of these relationships is to work with the table in Figure 3.3, holding sensitivity and specificity constant, changing prevalence, and calculating the resulting predictive values.

The effect of prevalence on positive predictive value, for a test with high sensitivity and specificity, is illustrated in Figure 3.7. When prevalence of disease in the population tested is relatively high—over several %—the test performs well. But at lower prevalences, the positive predictive value drops to nearly zero and the test is virtually useless for diagnosing disease.

Table 3.2

Effect of Prevalence on Predictive Value: Positive Predictive Value of Prostatic Acid Phosphatase for Prostatic Cancer (Sensitivity = 70%, Specificity = 90%) in Various Clinical Settiings*

Setting	Prevalence (Cases/100,000)	Postive Predictive Value (%)
General population	35	0.4
Men, age 75 or greater	500	5.6
Clinically suspicious prostatic nodule	50,000	93.0

* From: Watson RA, Tang DB. *N Engl J Med*, 1980; 303:497–499.

Example—The predictive value of prostatic acid phosphatase for carcinoma of the prostate was studied using several different prevalences, corresponding to various clinical situations (Table 3.2). In the general population, where the prevalence of prostatic carcinoma is estimated to be 35/100,000 only 0.4% of men with positive test results actually have cancer. In high risk men (over 75 years old, where it is estimated that 500/100,000 would have cancer), 5.6% of positive tests represent cancer. In other words, if prostatic acid phosphatase were used as a screening test, even for these high risk men, 18 men with positive tests would have to be evaluated with additional tests in order to find one with cancer. However, when there is a strong clinical suspicion of malignancy, because a nodule is felt, half of such men have prostatic cancer. In this situation, 93% of men with a positive test will have prostatic cancer (4).

One reason why prevalence is often more important than sensitivity and specificity in determining predictive value is that prevalence commonly varies over a wider range. By current standards, clinicians are not particularly interested in tests with sensitivities and specificities much below 50%, but if both sensitivity and specificity are 99%, the test is considered a great one. In other words, in practical terms sensitivity and specificity rarely vary more than two-fold. Prevalence of disease, however, can vary over a thousand fold in various clinical settings. In Table 3.2, the prevalence of prostatic cancer varied from 35/100,000 to 50,000/100,000.

Implications for the Medical Literature

Published descriptions of diagnostic tests often include, in addition to sensitivity and specificity, some conclusions about the interpretation of a positive or negative test (that is, predictive value). This is done, quite rightly, in order to provide information directly useful to clinicians. But the data for these publications are often gathered in university teaching hospitals where the prevalence of serious disease is relatively high. As a result, statements about predictive value in the medical literature may be misleading when the test is applied in less highly selected settings. What is worse, authors often compare the performance of a test in a number of patients known to have the disease and an equal number of patients without the disease. This is an efficient way to describe sensitivity and specificity. However, any reported positive predictive value from such studies may be falsely elevated because it has been determined for a group of patients in which the prevalence of disease is about 50%. Such a prevalence rarely corresponds to naturally occurring group of patients to which the test might be applied in practice (although such high prevalences can occur, as illustrated in Table 3.2).

STATISTICAL SIGNIFICANCE

Often the authors of a paper describing the properties of a diagnostic test point out that there is a statistically significant difference in the test results between those who do and do not have the disease in question. (Statistical significance is taken up in detail in Chapter 9.) It is important not to misinterpret such a statement as meaning that the test is really valuable for the purpose of assigning a diagnosis. Rather, it means that the observed differences between the test values for diseased and non-diseased individuals in the particular study being reported are unlikely to have arisen by chance alone. The overlap between test results in diseased and non-diseased individuals, however, still may be so great as to compromise the test's usefulness for clinical diagnosis.

Example—Figure 3.8 illustrates how a test, in this case plasma digoxin concentration, can be associated with a highly statistically significant difference between diseased and non-diseased subjects, yet be of limited value in practice. A statistically significant difference exists between the digoxin levels of patients known to be toxic, as compared to those who are non-toxic. But except for extremely high or low levels it is not possible to choose a level at which a clinically useful distinction can be made between toxic and non-toxic patients. For example, if a level of 2.0 ng/ml were chosen, 20 of 22 toxic patients would be correctly called toxic (sensitivity 91%), but 18 of 86 non-toxic patients would also be considered to have an abnormal digoxin level (specificity = 79%). The positive predictive value in this case is 53% and is not particularly useful. Of course, the positive predictive value would change if the prevalence of toxicity among the patients tested changed. In the example cited, the prevalence of toxicity was 22/108 or 20%, reflecting the particular set of patients selected for study. The prevalence of digitalis toxicity might be entirely different in other settings (5).

SUMMARY

Diagnostic test performance is judged by comparing the results of the test to the presence of disease in a four-cell table. All four cells must be filled. When estimating the sensitivity and specificity of a new diagnostic test from information in the medical literature, the clinician should examine the gold standard against which the accuracy of the test is compared. The diseased and non-diseased subjects both should resemble the kinds of patients for whom the test might be useful in practice. In addition, the final diagnosis should not influence the interpretation of the test results, or vice versa.

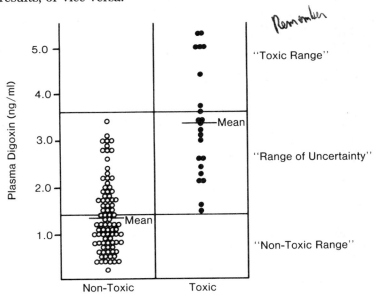

Figure 3.8. Example of Statistical versus Clinical Difference. Plasma Digoxin Concentrations and Digoxin Toxicity. (Redrawn from: Evered DC, Chapman C. *Br Heart J*, 1971; 33:540–545.)

The predictive value of a test is the characteristic most relevant to clinicians who interpret test results. It is determined not only by sensitivity and specificity of the test, but also by the prevalence of the disease, which may change from setting to setting.

Finally, test results may distinguish statistically between categories of patients, without being useful clinically.

Suggested Readings

Feinstein AR. Chapter 15: On the Sensitivity, Specificity and Discrimination of Diagnostic Tests. Clinical Biostatistics. St. Louis: C.V. Mosby Co., 1977.

Griner PF, Mayewski RJ, Mushlin AI, Greenland P. Selection and interpretation of diagnostic tests and procedures: Principles and applications. *Ann Intern Med* 1981; 94:553–600.

Ransohoff DF, Feinstein AR. Problems of spectrum and bias in evaluating the efficacy of diagnostic tests. *N Engl J Med* 1978; 299:926–930.

Department of Clinical Epidemiology and Biostatistics, McMaster University Health Sciences Centre. Clinical Epidemiology Rounds. How to read clinical journals: II. To learn about a diagnostic test. *Can Med Assoc J*, 1981; 124:703–710.

Sackett DL. Clinical diagnosis and the clinical laboratory. *Clin Invest Med*, 1978; 1:37–43.

References

1. Bartrum RJ, Crow HC, Foote SR. Ultrasonic and radiographic cholecystography. *N Engl J Med*, 1977; 296:538–541.
2. Cooperberg PL, Burhenne HJ. Real-time ultrasonography: diagnostic technique of choice in calculous gallbladder disease. *N Engl J Med*, 1980; 302:1277–1279.
3. Malcom ID, Flegel KM, Katz M. Vacualization of the neutrophil in bacteremia. *Arch Intern Med*, 1979; 139:675–676.
4. Watson RA, Tang DB. The predictive value of prostatic acid phosphatase as a screening test for prostatic cancer. *N Engl J Med*, 1980; 303:497–499.
5. Evered DC, Chapman C. Plasma digoxin concentrations and digoxin toxicity in hospital patients. *Br Heart J*, 1971; 33:540–545.

chapter

4

Diagnostic Strategies

Chapter 3 dealt with properties of individual diagnostic tests. This chapter will focus on strategies that clinicians use in order to increase the efficiency of the diagnostic process: increasing the prevalence of disease before employing tests and using many tests together. We also will discuss strategies for the particular situation when diagnostic tests are used to screen for disease.

INCREASING THE PREVALENCE OF DISEASE

Considering the relationship between the predictive value of a test and prevalence, it is obviously to the physician's advantage to apply diagnostic tests to patients with an increased likelihood of having the disease being sought. There are a variety of ways in which the probability of a disease can be increased before using a diagnostic test.

Referral Process

The referral process is one of the most common ways in which the probability of disease is increased. Teaching hospital wards, clinics, and emergency departments are frequently involved in this referral process, both because outside physicians formally refer patients and because patients informally refer themselves. The process increases the chance of significant disease underlying patients' complaints. Therefore, relatively more aggressive use of diagnostic tests might be justified in these settings.

In primary care practice, on the other hand, or among patients without complaints, the chance of finding disease is considerably smaller and tests should be used more sparingly.

Example—While practicing in a military clinic, one of the authors saw hundreds of people with headache, rarely ordered diagnostic tests, and never encountered a patient with a severe underlying cause of headache. (It is unlikely that important conditions were missed because the clinic was virtually the only source of medical care for these patients and prolonged follow-up was available.) However, during the first week back in a medical residency, a patient visiting his hospital's emergency department because of a headache similar to the ones managed in the military was found to have a cerebellar abscess!

Because clinicians may work at different extremes of the prevalence spectrum at various times in their clinical practices, they should bear in mind that the intensity of diagnostic evaluation may need to be adjusted to suit the specific situation.

Selected Demographic Groups

In a given setting, physicians can increase the yield of diagnostic tests by applying them to selected demographic groups known to be at higher risk for a disease. A man of 65 is 15 times more likely to have coronary artery disease as the cause of atypical chest pain than a woman of 30; thus, a particular diagnostic test for coronary disease, the electrocardiographic stress test, is less useful in confirming the diagnosis in the younger woman than in the older man (1). Similarly, a sickle test would obviously have a higher positive predictive value among blacks than among whites.

Specifics of the Clinical Situation

The specifics of the clinical situation are clearly the strongest influence on the decision to order tests. Symptoms, signs, or even vague "clinical impressions" all raise or lower the probability of finding a disease. For example, a woman with pleurisy is more likely to have had a pulmonary embolus if she has tenderness and swelling in her leg and if she is on oral contraceptives than if she has none of these features. As a result, an abnormal lung scan is more likely to represent a pulmonary embolus in such a woman than in persons with pleurisy, but without any particular reason for having an embolus.

Magnitude of the Effect of Prevalence

The value of applying specific diagnostic tests to persons more likely to have a particular illness is intuitively obvious to most doctors. Nevertheless, with the increasing availability of diagnostic tests, it is easy to adopt a less selective approach when ordering tests. However, the less selective the approach, the lower the prevalence of the disease is likely to be and the lower will be the positive predictive value of the test.

The magnitude of this effect can be larger than most of us might think.

Example—Factors which influence the interpretation of an abnormal electrocardiographic stress test are illustrated in Figure 4.1. It shows that the positive predictive value for coronary artery disease associated with an abnormal test can vary from 1.7 to 99.8%, depending on age, symptoms, and the degree of abnormality of the test. Thus, an exercise test in an asymptomatic 35-year-old man showing 1 mm ST segment depression will be a false positive test in over 98% of cases. The same test result in a 60-year-old man with typical angina by history will be associated with coronary artery disease in over 90% of cases (1).

Because of this effect, physicians must interpret similar test results differently in different clinical situations. In the previous example, a

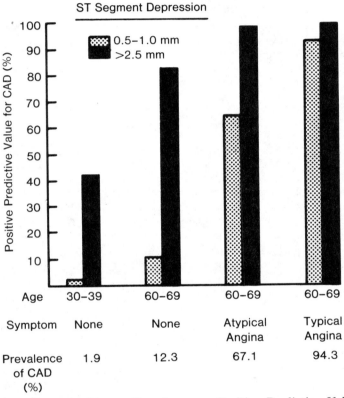

Figure 4.1. Effect of Disease Prevalence on Positive Predictive Value of a Diagnostic Test. Likelihood of Coronary Artery Disease (CAD) in Men According to Age, Symptom, and Depression of the ST Segment on Electrocardiogram. Prevalence is for Age and Symptom Groups. (Data from: Diamond GA, Forrester JS. *N Engl J Med*, 1979; 300:1350–1358.)

stress test in an asymptomatic 35-year-old man may be appropriate to confirm the absence of coronary artery disease, but usually will be misleading if it is used to search for unsuspected disease, as has been done among joggers, airline pilots, and business executives. The opposite applies to the 65-year-old man with typical angina. In this case, the test may be helpful in confirming disease but not in excluding disease. The test is most useful in intermediate situations, in which prevalence is neither very high nor very low. For example, a 60-year-old man with atypical chest pain has a 67% chance of coronary artery disease before stress testing (Figure 4.1); but afterwards, with greater than 2.5 mm ST segment depression, he has a 99% probability of coronary disease.

Because prevalence of disease is such a powerful determinant of how useful a diagnostic test for disease will be, clinicians must consider the probability of disease before ordering a test. The major means of doing so is by accurately interpreting the clinical context through careful observation during the history and physical examination. In an age when laboratory technology offers promise for solving complex diagnostic problems, we must still depend on medicine's oldest process—astute clinical observation.

MULTIPLE TESTS

Because clinicians commonly use imperfect diagnostic tests, with less than 100% sensitivity and specificity, a single test frequently results in a probability of disease which is neither very high nor very low—for example, somewhere between 10% and 90%. Usually it is not acceptable to stop the diagnostic process at such a point. Would a physician or patient be satisfied with the conclusion that the patient has a 50/50 chance of having carcinoma of the colon? Or that an asymptomatic 35-year-old man with 2.5 mm ST segment depression on a stress test has a 42% chance of coronary artery disease (Figure 4.1)? The physician is ordinarily bound to raise or lower the probability of disease substantially in such situations—unless, of course, the diagnostic possibilities are all trivial, nothing could be done about the result, or the risk of proceeding further is prohibitive. When these exceptions do not apply, the doctor will want to proceed with further tests.

When multiple tests are performed and all are positive or all are negative, the interpretation is straightforward. All too often, however, some are positive and others are negative. Interpretation is then more complicated. This section will discuss the principles by which multiple tests are interpreted.

Multiple tests can be applied in two general ways (Figure 4.2). They can be used in *parallel*, i.e., all at once, and a positive result of any test considered evidence for disease. Or they can be done *serially*, i.e., consecutively, each based on the results of the previous test. For serial testing, all tests must give a positive result for the diagnosis to be made, since the diagnostic process is stopped when a negative result is obtained.

Parallel Tests

Physicians usually order tests in parallel when rapid assessment is necessary, as in hospitalized or emergency patients, or ambulatory patients who cannot return easily because they have come from a long distance for evaluation.

Multiple tests in parallel increase the sensitivity, and therefore the negative predictive value, for a given disease prevalence above those of each individual test. On the other hand, specificity and positive predictive value are lowered. That is, disease is less likely to be missed (parallel testing is probably one reason referral centers seem to diagnose disease that local physicians miss), but false positive diagnoses are also more likely to be made (thus, the propensity for over-diagnosing in such centers as well). These relationships are demonstrated in Table 4.1.

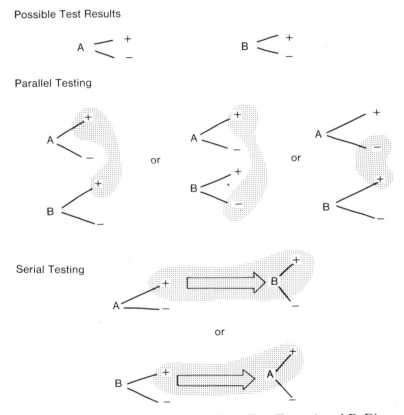

Figure 4.2. Parallel and Serial Testing Using Two Tests, A and B. Diagnoses Made According to Various Combinations of Test Results (Shown by *Stippled Areas*).

Parallel testing is particularly useful when the clinician is faced with the need for a very sensitive test but has available only two or more relatively insensitive ones. By using the tests in parallel, the net effect is a more sensitive diagnostic strategy. The price, however, is evaluation or treatment of some patients without the disease.

Example—Diagnosis of deep vein thrombosis in the leg remains a difficult clinical challenge. The most accurate test (i.e., gold standard) is venography involving injection of radiographic dye into the venous system of the leg. But venography is both expensive and somewhat risky; many physicians are reluctant to use it in every patient suspected of having deep vein thrombophlebitis.

As an alternative approach, two less accurate tests were used in parallel: impedance plethysmography and leg scanning after an injection of ^{125}I fibrinogen. Although neither test alone was as sensitive and specific as venography, using the two together achieved a sensitivity of 94% and a specificity of 91% (Figure 4.3).

In this situation, a parallel testing strategy could improve patient care by providing an accurate, safe, and less expensive alternative to venography (2).

Serial Testing

Physicians most commonly use serial testing strategies in clinical situations where rapid assessment of patients is not required, such as in office practices and hospital clinics in which ambulatory patients are followed over time. Serial testing is also used when some of the tests are expensive or risky, these tests being employed only after simpler and

Table 4.1

Effect of Parallel and Serial Testing on Sensitivity, Specificity, and Predictive Value of Test Combinations

Test	Sensitivity (%)	Specificity (%)	Positive Predictive Value* (%)	Negative Predictive Value* (%)
A	80	60	33	92
B	90	90	69	97
A or B (Parallel)	98	54	35	99
A and B (Serial)	72	96	82	93

* For 20% prevalence

safer tests suggest the presence of disease. Serial testing leads to less laboratory utilization than parallel testing because additional evaluation is contingent on prior test results. However, serial testing takes more time because additional tests are ordered as the results of previous ones become available.

Serial testing maximizes specificity and positive predictive value, but lowers sensitivity and the negative predictive value (Table 4.1). One ends up surer that positive test results represent disease, but runs an increased risk that disease will be missed.

Serial testing is particularly useful when none of the individual tests available to a clinician is highly specific. For example, of the three enzyme tests for myocardial infarction listed in Table 4.2, none is very specific. As a result, many patients might be falsely diagnosed as having suffered a myocardial infarction if one or the other were used alone. By using the three together, specificity is increased. Sensitivity, however, is somewhat decreased.

If a physician is going to use two tests in series, everything else being equal, the test with the highest specificity should be used first. Table 4.3

shows the effect of sequence on serial testing. Test A is more specific than test B (while B is more sensitive than A). By using A first, fewer patients are subjected to both tests, even though equal numbers of diseased patients are diagnosed, regardless of the sequence of tests.

Venography Results

	Positive	Negative	
Either or Both Positive	81	10	91
Both Negative	5	104	109
	86	114	200

IPG or Scan Results

Sensitivity: 81/86   = 94%
Specificity: 104/114 = 91%
+PV: 81/91   = 89%
−PV: 104/109 = 95%

Figure 4.3.   Example of Parallel Testing in the Diagnosis of Deep Vein Thrombosis: Comparing the Combination of Leg Scanning and Impedance Plethysmography (IPG) to Venography. Sensitivity of each procedure alone was 74%. +PV = Positive Predictive Value. −PV = Negative Predictive Value. (From: Hull R, Hirsh J, Sackett DL, Powers P, Turpie AGG, Walker I. *N Engl J Med*, 1977; 296:1497–1500.)

Table 4.2
Increasing Specificity with Serial Testing: Serum Enzymes in Diagnosing Myocardial Infarction*

Enzyme Test	Sensitivity (%)	Specificity (%)
CPK	96	57
SGOT	91	74
LDH	87	91
CPK, SGOT, and LDH	78	95

* From: Galen RS, Gambino SR. Beyond Normality: The Predictive Value and Efficiency of Medical Diagnoses. Chapter 6. New York: John Wiley & Sons, 1975.

Assumption of Independence

When multiple tests are used, it is often assumed that the additional information contributed by each test is independent of that already available from the preceding ones—that is, the next test does not simply duplicate known information. In fact, this assumption underlies the entire approach to predictive value we have discussed. The assumption is likely to be correct when a manifestation of disease changes with time, as when

Table 4.3
Effect of Sequence in Serial Testing: A Then B versus B Then A*

Prevalence of Disease

Number of patients tested	1000
Number of patients with disease	200 (20% prevalence)

Sensitivity and Specificity of Tests

Test	Sensitivity	Specificity
A	80	90
B	90	80

Sequence of Testing

Begin with Test A

	Disease +	Disease −	
A +	160	80	240
A −	40	720	760
	200	800	1000

Begin with Test B

	Disease +	Disease −	
B +	180	160	340
B −	20	640	660
	200	800	1000

240 Patients Retested with B

	Disease +	Disease −	
B +	144	16	160
B −	16	64	80
	160	80	240

340 Patients Retested with A

	Disease +	Disease −	
A +	144	16	160
A −	46	144	180
	180	160	340

* Note that in both sequences the same number of patients are identified as diseased (160), and the same number of true positives (144) are identified. But when Test A (with the higher specificity) is used first, fewer patients are retested. The lower sensitivity of Test A does not adversely affect the final result.

stool is tested for occult blood repeatedly on the belief that an occult malignancy bleeds intermittently. Independence of tests also is likely if the tests are measuring different phenomena. In the example of plethysmography and leg scanning for diagnosing deep vein thrombophlebitis (pages 63–64), there is evidence that plethysmography picks up thromboses in the thigh, whereas leg scanning is better at finding thromboses in the calf. Thus, these tests may complement each other.

However, it seems unlikely that multiple tests for most diseases are truly independent of one another. If the assumption that the tests are completely independent is wrong, calculation of the probability of disease from several tests would tend to overestimate the tests' value.

SCREENING FOR DISEASE

We have been discussing the use of diagnostic tests in the care of sick patients, or at least for patients with specific complaints. However, diagnostic tests are also used on well patients—to identify risk factors or find disease early in its course and, by intervening, keep patients well. Such activity is often referred to as preventive health care, the routine physical, or the periodic health examination. Periodic health examinations constitute a large portion of clinical practice; in a national survey of ambulatory care, they accounted for almost one-fifth of office practice (3). Physicians must be able, therefore, to decide about the content of the periodic health examination. They must be prepared to answer such questions as, "Why do I have to get a pap smear again this year, doctor?" or "My neighbor gets a chest X-ray every year; why aren't you ordering one for me?"

Many of the strategies and principles already discussed apply to screening for disease. Several additional principles are outlined in this section. Although discussed in the context of the periodic health examination, many of these principles are important in other clinical situations as well, although in given clinical circumstances one or another may deserve more emphasis.

Definitions

Screening has been defined as "the presumptive identification of unrecognized disease or defect by the application of tests, examinations, or other procedures which can be applied rapidly." Furthermore, "screening tests sort out apparently well persons who have a disease from those who probably do not. A screening test is not intended to be diagnostic. Persons with positive or suspicious findings must be referred to their physicians for diagnosis and treatment" (4).

When screening tests are applied to large unselected populations, the process is called *mass screening*. Blood pressure measurements on passers-by in a shopping mall are an example of mass screening. Clinicians, on the other hand, use screening tests in a different context. Their concern about unrecognized disease is not so much for the population at large but for their own patients. *Case finding* occurs when clinicians search for disease with screening tests among their own patients, who are consulting for unrelated symptoms.

The distinction between mass screening and case finding is subtle but important. In the shopping mall, those examining the patient have no personal responsibility for following up abnormal results with appropriate diagnosis and treatment. Instead, the patient is referred to his or her doctor; many studies have shown inadequate follow-up among people with abnormalities found in mass screening. On the other hand, in case finding, the clinician has the explicit responsibility for follow-up of abnormal results. If the clinician is not committed to further investigation of abnormal results, the test should not be performed in the first place.

Orientation: Diseases, then Tests

When considering which screening tests to perform routinely on well patients, a decision first must be made as to which medical problems or diseases should be sought. This statement is so straightforward that it would seem unnecessary. But the fact is, many tests are suggested without any clear understanding of what is being sought. For instance, a urinalysis is frequently ordered by physicians performing routine check-ups on their patients. But a urinalysis might be used to search for any number of medical problems, including diabetes, asymptomatic urinary tract infections, and renal calculi. It is necessary to decide which if any of these conditions is worth screening for before undertaking the test (Table 4.4).

In order to decide whether a disease should be sought in a periodic health examination, the first question which must be answered relates to treatment of the condition. Is there an effective treatment if the medical problem is found early? If not, it is not worth searching for the medical problem in periodic health examinations regardless of how easily it may be found. This principle is illustrated by a study of the use of chest X-rays to screen for lung cancer. People who were screened every six months with X-ray examinations and treated promptly if cancer was found did no better than those not examined; at five years less than 10% of patients with lung cancer were alive in either group (5). Early detection and treatment, therefore, did not help patients with lung cancer.

Effectiveness of treatment is covered in detail in Chapter 8. In the context of screening, for a treatment to be effective: 1) the treatment itself must work (efficacy), 2) patients must accept the treatment (patient compliance), and 3) the treatment must be applied early enough in the course of illness to prevent untoward sequelae, i.e., there must be sufficient lead time.

Lead time is the period of time between when a medical condition can be found by screening and when it ordinarily would have been diagnosed because an individual experienced symptoms and sought medical care (Figure 4.4). Lead time for a given disease is dependent on both the biologic rate of progression of the disease and the ability of the screening test to detect early disease. When lead time is very short, as is presently the case with lung cancer, the treatment of medical conditions picked up on screening is likely to be no more effective than treatment after symptoms appear.

A second question to be answered is how severe is the medical condition, in terms of the mortality, morbidity and suffering caused by it. Only conditions posing threats to life or health should be sought. Again, this statement appears straightforward, but sometimes it is not. For instance, the health consequences of asymptomatic bacteriuria are still unclear. We do not know if asymptomatic bacteriuria causes renal failure and/or hypertension. Even so, bacteriuria is a very common condition which is frequently sought in periodic health examinations. The severity of a medical condition is determined primarily by its risk or prognosis (discussed in Chapters 6 and 7).

Table 4.4
Criteria for Deciding whether a Medical Condition should be Sought During Periodic Health Examinations

1. If the condition is found, how effective is the ensuing treatment in terms of:
   Efficacy
   Patient compliance
   Lead time
2. How great is the burden of suffering caused by the condition in terms of:
   Mortality
   Disability
   Discomfort
   Financial costs
3. How good is the screening procedure in terms of:

Sensitivity	Cost
Specificity	Safety
Simplicity	Acceptability

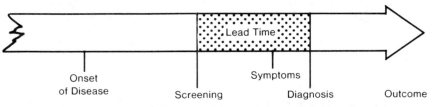

Figure 4.4. Lead Time Gained by Early Diagnosis during Screening.

In sum, the two most important criteria for deciding whether a medical condition should be sought in a periodic health examination are its treatability and its severity.

Test Criteria

With appropriate answers to the previous two questions, we can turn to criteria for the test itself. When considering the properties of the test, it should be borne in mind that:

1. The test should be sensitive and specific.

The very nature of searching for disease in asymptomatic people means the prevalence of a particular disease will usually be very low, even among "high risk" groups selected for age, sex, and other characteristics. Therefore, the positive predictive value of screening tests is likely to be low regardless of how specific a given test might be. A clinician who wants to practice preventive care by performing periodic health examinations on his patients, therefore, must accept the fact that he will have to work up many patients who will not have disease.

2. The test must be simple and cheap.

An ideal screening test should take only a few minutes to perform, require minimum preparation by the patient, require no special appointments, and be inexpensive.

Simple, quick examinations, such as blood pressure determinations, are ideal screening tests. Conversely, complicated diagnostic tests such as barium enemas which require special diet, an X-ray appointment, bowel preparation and discomfort during the procedure, may be reasonable in patients with symptoms and clinical indications, but are clearly unacceptable as screening tests. Other tests, such as visual field testing for the detection of glaucoma and audiograms for the detection of hearing loss, fall between these two extremes. If done carefully, such tests, although not as difficult as barium enemas, are probably too complex to be used as screening tests.

The financial "cost" of the test depends not only on the cost of (or charge for) the procedure itself but also on the cost of subsequent evaluations performed on patients with positive test results. Thus, sensitivity, specificity, and predictive value impact on cost. Cost is also affected by whether the test requires a special visit to the physician. Screening tests performed while the patient is seeing his or her physician for other reasons (as is frequently the case with blood pressure measurements) are much cheaper for patients than tests requiring special visits, extra time off from work and additional transportation.

3. The test must be very safe.

Although it is reasonable and ethical to accept certain risks for diagnostic tests applied to sick patients seeking help for specific complaints, it is quite another matter to subject presumably well people to such risks. Thus, although sigmoidoscopy using a rigid sigmoidoscope is hardly thought of as a "dangerous" procedure when used on patients with gastrointestinal complaints, some reviewers have suggested it is too dangerous to use as a screening procedure because of the possibility of bowel perforation. In fact, it has been estimated that if sigmoidoscopy were used to screen for colorectal cancer, as many as four perforations would occur for every cancer found (6).

4. The test must be acceptable to both patients and practitioners.

The importance of this criterion is illustrated by experience with tests for early cervical cancer and early colon cancer. It turns out that women at greatest risk for cervical cancer are least likely to get routine pap smears. The same problem holds true for colorectal cancer. Studies indicate there is a strong reluctance among asymptomatic North Americans to submit to periodic examinations of their lower gastrointestinal tracts—a finding which should be no surprise to any of us!

Table 4.5 illustrates the problem of patient acceptance of screening for colorectal cancer. People who were attending a colorectal cancer screening clinic were very cooperative; they were willing to collect stool samples, smear the samples on guaiac-impregnated paper slides, and mail the slides to their doctors for chemical testing. Less selected patients, however, were less willing to participate. Retired persons, who were at greatest risk for colorectal cancer because of their age, were least willing to be screened.

The acceptability of the test to clinicians is a criterion usually overlooked by all but the ones performing the test. After one large and well-conducted study on the usefulness of screening, sigmoidoscopy was abandoned because the physicians performing the procedure—gastroenterol-

Table 4.5
Patient Acceptance of Screening Tests: Reported Response Rates for Returning Guaiac-impregnated Slides in Different Settings*

Setting	Participants Returning at Least one Slide (%)
Colorectal cancer screening program	85
Breast cancer screening program	70
American Association of Retired Persons chapter meetings	29

* From: Fletcher SW, Dauphinee WD. *Clin Invest Med* 1981; 4:23–31.

ogists, at that—found it too cumbersome and time-consuming to be justified by the yield (7). (Patient acceptance, 38%, was not good either.)

The "Labelling" Effect

The *labelling* effect describes the psychologic impact of test results or diagnosis on patients. Labelling effects have not been extensively studied, but the work which has been done suggests that test results can sometimes have important psychologic effects on patients.

Theoretically, a labelling effect can work in either a positive or negative direction. A positive labelling effect may occur when a patient is told that all the screening test results were normal. Most clinicians have heard such responses as, "Great, that means I can keep working for another year." If being given a clean bill of health promotes a continued positive attitude towards one's daily activities, a positive labelling effect has occurred.

On the other hand, being told that something is abnormal may have an adverse psychologic effect. In one study, steelworkers who were told for the first time that they had hypertension experienced a three-fold increase in absenteeism, an increase which could not be explained by the medical condition itself. The authors suggested that newly labelled patients "adopt the 'sick role' and treat themselves as more 'fragile' " (8). The potential for this negative labelling effect is particularly worrisome if it occurs among patients with false positive tests; and false positive tests are particularly likely when screening because of the low prevalence of disease. In such situations screening efforts might do more harm than good.

The Risk of a False Positive Result

The previous discussion applies to each of the individual screening tests a clinician might consider performing during a periodic health examination. However, most clinicians do not perform only one or two tests on patients presenting for routine check-ups. In one study, practicing internists believed that 57 different tests should be performed during periodic health examinations (9). Modern technology has fueled this

Table 4.6
Relation Between Number of Tests Ordered and % of Normal People with at Least one Abnormal Test Result*

No. of Tests	People with at Least one Abnormality (%)
1	5
5	23
20	64
100	99.4

* From: Sackett DL. *Clin Invest Med*, 1978; 1:37–43.

propensity to "cover all the bases." Automated blood tests allow physicians to order up to several dozen tests with a few checks in the appropriate boxes.

When the measurements of screening tests are expressed on interval scales (as most are) and when normal is defined by the range covered by 95% of the results (as is usual), the more tests the clinician orders, the greater the risk of a false positive result. In fact, as Table 4.6 shows, if the physician orders enough tests a new abnormality will be discovered in virtually all healthy patients.

Current Recommendations

The search for disease and risk factors in presumably healthy patients is far more complex than was once thought. Because of these complexities, current recommendations on the periodic health examination are quite different from those of the past. Several groups have recommended abandoning routine annual check-ups in favor of a selective approach in which the tests to be done depend on a person's age and sex (thus, increasing prevalence). They have also tended to recommend fewer tests than previously (thus, decreasing the percentage of patients with false positive results). They have turned their attention to the selection process for deciding what medical conditions should be sought. Finally, there is an increasing concern for clear delineation of the standards tests should meet before they are incorporated into periodic health examinations.

SUMMARY

Because prevalence of disease is a powerful determinant of the predictive value of diagnostic tests, clinicans can maximize the usefulness of diagnostic tests by applying them to groups of patients with increased prevalence of disease. Strategies for increasing prevalence include the referral process, selection of specific demographic groups, and the clinical context.

Multiple diagnostic tests can be applied in parallel, increasing the sensitivity and negative predictive value of tests, or serially, increasing the specificity and positive predictive value of diagnostic tests.

When employing tests during periodic health examinations, physicians must consider the effectiveness of treatment for each medical condition sought, the seriousness of the condition, and several characteristics of the tests: sensitivity, specificity, simplicity, expense, safety, acceptability, and labelling effects. The more tests the physician orders, the more likely an abnormality will be found in normal patients.

Suggested Readings

Galen RS, Gambino SR. Beyond Normality. The Predictive Value and Efficiency of Medical Diagnosis. New York: John Wiley & Sons, 1975.

McNeil BJ, Keeler E, Adelstein SJ. Primer on certain elements of medical decision making. *N Engl J Med*, 1975; 293:211–215.

Weinstein MC, Fineberg HV, Elstein AS, Frazier HS, Neuhauser D, Neutra RR, McNeil BJ. Clinical Decision Analysis. Chapters 4–6. Philadelphia: WB Saunders, 1980.

Wulff HR. Rational Diagnosis and Treatment. London: Blackwell Scientific Publications, 1976.

Sackett DL, Holland WW. Controversy in the detection of disease. *Lancet*, 1975; 2:357–359.

Spitzer WO (Chairman). Report of the Task Force on the Periodic Health Examination. *Can Med Assoc J*, 1979; 121:1193–1245.

ACS report on the cancer-related health checkup. *Ca* 1980; 30:194–240.

Romm FJ, Fletcher SW, Hulka BS. The periodic health examination: Comparison of recommendations and internists' performance. *South Med J*, 1981; 74:265–271.

References

1. Diamond GA, Forrester JS. Analysis of probability as an aid in the clinical diagnosis of coronary artery disease. *N Engl J Med*, 1979; 300:1350–1358.
2. Hull R, Hirsh J, Sackett DL, Powers P, Turpie AGG, Walker I. Combined use of leg scanning and impedance plethysmography in suspected venous thrombosis. An alternative to venography. *N Engl J Med*, 1977; 296:1497–1500.
3. National Center for Health Statistics. The National Ambulatory Medical Care Survey: 1973 Summary, United States, May 1973–April 1974. Rockville, Maryland:National Center for Health Statistics, 1975 (DHEW Publication No. (HRA) 76-1772).
4. Commission on Chronic Illness. Chronic Illness in the United States; Vol 1. Cambridge, Massachusetts:Harvard University Press, 1957.

5. Brett GZ. The value of lung cancer detection by six-monthly chest radiographs. *Thorax*, 1968; 23:414–420.

6. Frame PS, Carlson SJ. A critical review of periodic health screening using specific screening criteria: Part 2. Selected endocrine, metabolic and gastrointestinal diseases. *J Fam Pract*, 1975; 2:123–129.

7. Dales LG, Friedman GD, Collen MF. Evaluating periodic multiphasic health check-ups: A controlled trial. *J Chron Dis*, 1979; 32:385–404.

8. Haynes RB, Sackett DL, Taylor DW, Gibson ES, Johnson AL. Increased absenteeism from work after detection and labelling of hypertensive patients. *N Engl J Med*, 1978; 299:741–744.

9. Hulka BS, Romm FJ, Parkerson GR, Russell IT, Clapp NE, Johnson MS. Peer review in ambulatory care: Use of explicit criteria and implicit judgments. *Med Care*, 1979; 17(3, Supplement):1–73.

chapter

5

Frequency

In Chapter 1, we outlined the central questions facing clinicians as they care for patients. In this chapter, we will build a foundation for the evidence which clinicians use to guide their diagnostic and therapeutic decisions. Let us introduce the subject with a patient.

A 22-year-old presents with sore throat, fever, and malaise of two days duration. Further history indicates no exposure to sick individuals and no prior history of significant illness. Physical examination reveals a temperature of 38°C, an erythematous pharynx with whitish exudate and tonsillar enlargement, tender anterior cervical lymph nodes, and no other positive findings.

In planning further diagnosis and treatment, the clinician must deal with several questions:
1. How likely is the patient to have streptococcal pharyngitis?
2. If the patient has streptococcal infection, how likely is it to lead to something much more serious such as acute rheumatic fever or acute glomerulonephritis?
3. How likely is penicillin treatment to prevent rheumatic fever or glomerulonephritis?
4. If the patient is treated with penicillin, how likely is an important allergic reaction?

Depending on the answers to these questions, the physician may treat with penicillin right away, obtain a throat culture and await the result, or offer only symptomatic treatment. Each of these questions concerns the likelihood or commonness of a clinical event under certain circumstances.

The questions could all be recast so as to ask—"How frequently do streptococcal pharyngitis or rheumatic fever or penicillin allergic reactions occur under particular circumstances?"

The evidence required to manage this patient rationally, the likelihood or frequency of disease or outcomes, is, in general, the kind of evidence needed to answer most clinical questions. Decisions are guided by the commonness of things. Usually, they depend on the relative commonness of things under alternative circumstances: in the presence of a positive test versus a negative test, or after Treatment A versus Treatment B. Because the commonness of disease, improvement, deterioration, cure, or death forms the basis for answering most clinical questions, this chapter will examine measures of clinical frequency.

STRUCTURE OF MEASURES OF CLINICAL FREQUENCY

In general, clinically relevant measures of the frequency of events are fractions in which the numerator is the number of patients experiencing the outcome (cases) and the denominator is the number of people in whom the outcome could have occurred. Such fractions are of course proportions but, by common usage, are often referred to as "rates." As ex-students of physics, we recognize the incorrectness of this use of rate; but there seems to be little chance that it will disappear.

Prevalence and Incidence

In general, clinicians encounter two measures of commonness—prevalence and incidence.

A *prevalence* is the fraction (proportion) of a group possessing a clinical outcome at a given point in time and is measured by a single examination or survey of a group. An *incidence* is the fraction or proportion of a group initially free of the outcome which develops the outcome over a given period of time. As described later in this chapter and in greater detail in Chapter 6, incidence is measured by identifying a susceptible group of people (i.e., people free of the disease or the outcome) and examining them periodically over an interval of time so as to discover and count new cases which develop during the interval.

To illustrate the differences between prevalence and incidence, Figure 5.1 shows the occurrence of disease in a group of 100 individuals over the course of three years (1971, 1972, 1973).

Prevalences are measured by surveying the total population, some of whom are diseased, at a single point in time. At the beginning of 1971, there are four cases, so the prevalence at that point in time is 4/100. If all 100 individuals, including prior cases, are examined at the beginning of each year, one can compute the prevalence at those points in time. At the beginning of 1972, the prevalence is 5/100 because two of the pre-1971 cases lingered on into 1972 and two of the new cases developing in 1971 terminated (hopefully in a cure) before the examination at the start of 1972. Prevalences can be computed for each of the other two annual examinations and, assuming that none of the original 100 people died, moved away, or refused examination, these prevalences are 7/100 at the beginning of 1973 and 5/100 at the beginning of 1974.

To calculate the incidence of new cases developing in the population, we consider only the 96 individuals free of the disease at the beginning of 1971 and what happens to them over the next three years. Five new cases developed in 1971; six new cases developed in 1972; and five additional new cases developed in 1973. The three-year incidence of the disease is

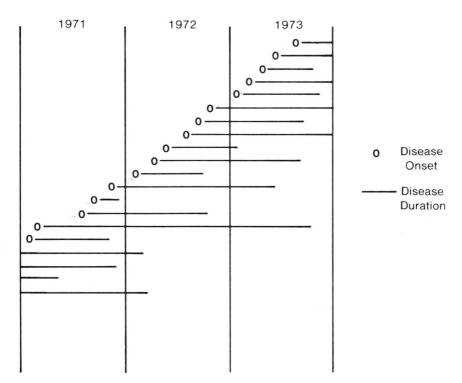

Figure 5.1. Occurrence of Disease in 100 Individuals from 1971–1973. Eighty individuals did not develop disease during the three years and do not appear in the figure.

all new cases developing in the three years (16) divided by the number of susceptible individuals at the beginning of the follow-up period (96), or 16/96 in three years. What would be the annual incidences for 1971, 1972, and 1973, respectively? Remembering to remove the previous cases from the denominator, the annual incidences would be 5/96 for 1971, 6/91 for 1972, and 5/85 for 1973.

Table 5.1 summarizes the characteristics of incidence and prevalence. Although the distinctions between the two seem clear, the literature is replete with misuses of the terms, particularly incidence (1). As we will point out, the distinctions are important.

MEASURING PREVALENCE AND INCIDENCE

Measuring Prevalence

Prevalent cases are discovered by surveying a group of people, some of whom are diseased at that point in time while others are healthy. The fraction or proportion of the group who are diseased (i.e., cases) constitutes the prevalence of the disease.

Such one-shot examinations or surveys of a population of individuals including cases and non-cases have been termed *prevalence* or *cross-sectional studies*. They are among the more common types of research designs reported in the medical literature, constituting approximately one-third of original articles in major medical journals.

Table 5.1

Characteristics of Incidence Rates and Prevalence Rates

Rate	Numerator	Denominator	Time	How Measured
Incidence	New cases occurring during the follow-up period in a group initially free of the disease.	All susceptible individuals present at the beginning of the follow-up period (often called the Population at Risk).	Duration of the follow-up period.	Cohort Study (see Chapter 6)
Prevalence	All cases counted on a single survey or examination of a group.	All individuals examined including cases and non-cases.	Single point in time.	Prevalence or cross-sectional study.

To illustrate prevalence, we will begin with an example of a typical prevalence study.

Example—Sixty-five autistic and psychotic children undergoing routine evaluation at a Child Psychiatric Study Unit were screened for genetic diseases. Three of the 65 were found to have positive ferric chloride urine tests and elevated blood phenylalanine levels diagnostic of phenylketonuria (prevalence = 3/65 = 4.6%).

The authors conclude that "urinary genetic screening should be a standard test for all children being evaluated for serious developmental disturbances of childhood" (2).

In this example, cases are children with phenylketonuria and the population is autistic and psychotic children seen at a child psychiatry center who were surveyed for phenylketonuria during a single examination.

The next example is less straightforward.

Example—In a study of the determinants of work loss in rheumatoid arthritis, twenty-five rheumatologists were asked to identify all patients with rheumatoid arthritis visiting their offices during a one-month period. Patients were eligible for the study only if they had been working at the time their arthritis was first manifest.

A total of 180 patients were eligible. They were interviewed regarding their present work status, and nearly 60% had given up their jobs because of their disease. Factors associated with work loss included the duration of the disease, and the control that the patient exercised over the nature or pace of job activities.

In this prevalence study, the population consists of rheumatoid arthritis patients working at the time of disease onset and receiving care from selected rheumatologists. The outcome or case whose prevalence was being measured was work loss. This is a prevalence study because the presence or absence of work loss was measured at a single point in time. Work losses were counted as long as they occurred anytime after the first presentation of the arthritis, which averaged 10 years before the survey, and persisted until the time of the survey (3).

Superficially, this example seems to report the occurrence of events over time. But it is a prevalence study too, because the outcome—work loss—was measured at one point in time, in a group of patients identified after the outcome had occurred.

In many prevalence studies, not only is the disease or outcome measured, but factors which are believed to be associated with the disease or outcome are also measured at the same time. In this example, a variety of characteristics for each patient—arthritis, social and work situation, and treatment—were measured in an effort to account for the presence or absence of work loss.

Measuring Incidence

In contrast to prevalence, incidence is measured by first identifying a population free of the event of interest, and then following them through time with periodic examinations for occurrences of the event. This process, called a cohort study, will be discussed in detail in Chapter 6.

Time

Every measure of disease frequency of necessity contains some indication of time. With measures of prevalence, time is assumed to be instantaneous, like a single frame from a motion picture. Prevalence depicts the situation at that point in time for each patient even though it may, in reality, have taken several weeks or months to collect observations on the various people in the group studied.

For incidence, time is the essence because it defines the interval during which susceptible subjects were monitored for the emergence of the event of interest. Two distinct approaches to the assessment of incidence are encountered in the medical literature.

One approach to incidence is to describe the number of new cases occurring in a fixed group of initially susceptible individuals followed for a defined interval of time.

Example—The death rate after acute respiratory failure complicating chronic respiratory disease was studied by observing the survival of 145 patients. After 1 year, 90 patients had died, for a death rate (incidence of death) of 90/145 = 62/100/year. After 5 years, the death rate was 122/145 = 84/100/5 years (4).

A second approach to incidence is to measure the number of new cases emerging in an ever-changing population, where subjects are under study and susceptible for varying lengths of time. Typical examples are clinical trials of chronic treatment in which eligible patients are enrolled over several years so that early enrollees are treated and followed longer than late enrollees. In an effort to keep the contribution of individual subjects commensurate with their follow-up interval, the denominator of the incidence measure in these studies is not persons at risk for a specific time period but person-time at risk of the event. An individual followed for 10 years without becoming a case contributes 10 person-years, while an individual followed for one year contributes only one person-year to the denominator. An incidence of this type is expressed as the number of new cases per total number of person-years at risk and is sometimes called an *incidence density.*

A disadvantage of the incidence density approach is that it lumps together different lengths of follow-up. A small number of patients followed for a long time can contribute as much to the denominator as a large number of patients followed for a short time. If these long follow-up patients are systematically different from short follow-up patients, the resulting incidence measures may be biased.

SOURCES OF BIAS IN PREVALENCE STUDIES

Interpreting Temporal Sequences

Prevalence studies are used to answer two kinds of questions. They are ideally suited for one. For the second, they are quick but inferior alternatives to cohort studies.

First, prevalence studies can be used to provide a quantitative description of the situation as it exists at that time. Questions relating to diagnosis (see Chapters 3 and 4) fit this category. We are usually interested in the ability of a diagnostic test to classify patients correctly at a single point in time, and a prevalence survey of an appropriate patient group fills the need perfectly. Similarly, the prevalence survey of disturbed children cited in the earlier example provided the kind of one-time diagnostic information needed to address the question of the value of screening for genetic diseases. The study would have been enhanced by similar screening of a relevant comparison group.

Second, prevalence can be used to study potentially causal relationships between various factors and a disease or outcome. However, disease and the possible factors responsible for the disease are measured simultaneously and so it is often unclear which came before the other. The time dimension is lost and if it is included in the interpretation it must be inferred. In contrast, studies of incidence do have a built-in sequence of events because possible causes of disease are measured initially, before disease has occurred. These relationships are illustrated in Figure 5.2.

The difficulties of interpretation that may result when temporal sequences must be inferred in a prevalence study can be illustrated by the example of work loss in rheumatoid arthritis. Because the possible causative factors (e.g., control over one's job) and outcome (work disability) were both measured after the fact, it is not possible to know whether the purported "causes" preceded the effects or followed them. It is implied that little control over one's job led to loss of job after the onset of arthritis. But it is also perfectly reasonable to conclude that patients who have lost their jobs will then believe that they had little control over that job. A cohort study of the same question would measure

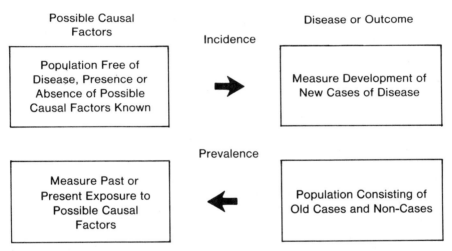

Figure 5.2. Temporal Relationship Between Possible Causal Factors and Disease: Incidence and Prevalence.

feelings of control over one's job while the subjects were employed and then follow them over time to see who stopped working. With this approach, there would have been no question about the sequence of events.

Therefore, an important limitation of prevalence studies of cause is that one can rarely be certain of the sequence of events.

Old Versus New Cases

The difference between cases found in the numerator of incidences and of prevalences is illustrated in Figure 5.3. In a cohort study, most new cases can be ascertained if a susceptible population is followed carefully through time. On the other hand, prevalence surveys include old as well as new cases, and they include only those cases that are available at the time of a single examination—that is, they identify only cases which happen to be both active (i.e., diagnosable) and alive at the time of the survey. Obviously, prevalences will be dominated by those patients who are able to survive their disease without losing its manifestations.

In many situations, the kinds of cases included in the numerator of an incidence are quite different from the kinds of cases included in the numerator of a prevalence. The differences may influence how the rates are interpreted.

Prevalence is affected by the average duration of disease. Rapidly fatal episodes of the disease would be included in an incidence but most would be missed by a prevalence survey. For example, 25–40% of all deaths from

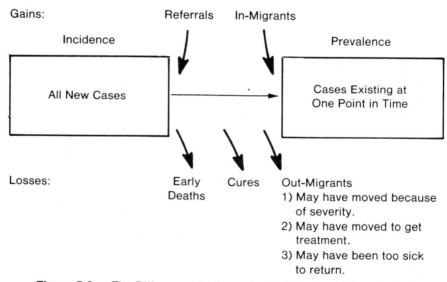

Figure 5.3.   The Differences in Cases for Incidence and Prevalence.

coronary heart disease occur within 24 hours of the onset of symptoms in individuals with no prior evidence of disease. A prevalence survey would, therefore, underestimate new cases of coronary heart disease. On the other hand, diseases of long duration are well represented in prevalence surveys, even if their incidence is low. For example, although the incidence of Crohn's disease is only about 2–7/100,000/year, its prevalence is over 100/100,000, reflecting the chronic nature of the disease (5).

Prevalence surveys can also selectively include more severe cases of disease, ones that are particularly sustained and obtrusive. For example, patients with rheumatoid arthritis who ceased work and then resumed their jobs would not be counted as cases in the example described previously. Similarly, patients with recurrent but controllable illnesses such as congestive heart failure or depression may be well at a given point in time, and therefore might not be discovered on a single examination. Unremitting disease, on the other hand, is less likely to be overlooked and, therefore, would contribute disproportionately to the pool of cases assembled by a prevalence survey.

The following is an example of the relationship between prevalence and severity of disease.

Example—During a long-term follow-up study of 539 women with atypical cervical cytologic smears, it was possible to compare progression of cytologic changes in incident and prevalent cases. Of women whose initial smears were atypical (prevalent cases), 41% progressed to more malignant stages on repeat examinations. Conversely, only 18% of women showing cervical atypia after a previous normal examination (incident cases) progressed to more malignant stages.

In this study, prevalent cases demonstrated more severe disease, probably because the duration of their atypia was longer (6).

Relationship Between Incidence, Prevalence, and Duration of Disease

As described previously anything which increases the duration of the clinical findings in a patient will increase the chance that that patient will be identified in a prevalence study. The relationship between incidence and prevalence and duration of disease has been approximated by the expression:

$$\text{Prevalence} \approx \text{Incidence} \times \text{Average Duration of the Disease}$$

Example—Table 5.2 shows approximate annual incidence and prevalence rates for asthma. Incidence falls with increasing age, illustrating the fact that the disease arises primarily in childhood. But prevalence stays fairly stable over the entire age span, indicating that asthma tends to be chronic and is especially chronic among older individuals. Also, because the pool of prevalent cases does not increase in size, about the same number of patients are recovering from their asthma as new patients are acquiring it.

If we use the formula (Prevalence = Incidence × Average Duration), we can determine that asthma has an average duration of 10 years. When the duration of asthma is determined for each age category by dividing the prevalences by the incidence, it is apparent that the duration of asthma increases with increasing age. This reflects the clinical observation that childhood asthma often clears with time whereas adult asthma tends to be more chronic.

INTERPRETING MEASURES OF CLINICAL FREQUENCY

In order to make sense out of prevalences and incidences, the first step is a careful evaluation of the numerator and denominator. Two questions serve to guide this evaluation: what is a case, and what is the population?

What is a "Case"?—Defining the Numerator

Up to this point, the term case has been used to indicate a disease or outcome whose frequency is of interest. Classically, prevalence and incidence refer to the frequency of a disease among groups of people and accordingly have been designated measures of disease frequency. However, clinical problems often require evidence of the frequency of disease manifestations such as symptoms, signs, or laboratory abnormalities or the frequency of disease end-points such as death, disability, symptomatic improvement, etc.

To interpret rates, it is necessary to know the basis upon which a case is defined, because the criteria used to define a case can strongly affect rates.

Example—One simple way to identify a case is to ask people whether they have a certain condition. How does this method compare to more rigorous methods? In the Commission on Chronic Illness study, the prevalences of various conditions, as determined by personal interview in the home, were compared to the prevalences as determined by physician examination of the same individuals. Table 5.3 illustrates the ratio of the interview prevalences to the clinical examination prevalences for various conditions.

The data illustrate that these two methods of defining a case can generate very

Table 5.2
The Relationships Among Incidence, Prevalence and Duration of Disease. Asthma in the United States

Age	Annual Incidence	Prevalence	Duration = $\dfrac{\text{Prevalence}}{\text{Annual Incidence}}$
0–5	6/1000	29/1000	4.8 years
6–16	3/1000	32/1000	10.7 years
17–44	2/1000	26/1000	13.0 years
45–64	1/1000	33/1000	33.0 years
65+	0	36/1000	
	3/1000	30/1000	10.0 years

different estimates of prevalence, and in different directions, depending on the condition (7).

In the example cited, common sense suggests that clinical evaluation would provide more valid estimates of the frequency of cases than the report of people themselves. But even when clinical evaluation by experienced clinicians is used to diagnose a case, problems can occur.

Example—Three cardiologists examined 57 men with chest pain to determine which had angina pectoris. All three physicians agreed that 17 men (30%) did have angina and that 26 (46%) did not. However, the cardiologists could not agree about 14 (25%) of the men. Depending on how their disagreement is resolved, the prevalence of angina in this group of men with chest pain could be anywhere from 30–55% (8).

For some conditions, broadly accepted, explicit diagnostic criteria are available. The American Rheumatism Association criteria for rheumatoid arthritis (Table 5.4) are an example (9). These criteria demonstrate the extraordinary specificity required to define reliably so common a disease as rheumatoid arthritis. They also illustrate a trade-off between rigorous definition and clinical reality. If only "classic" cases were included in a rate, most patients who would ordinarily be considered to have the disease would not be included. On the other hand, including "probable" cases could overestimate the true rate of disease.

What is the Population?—Defining the Denominator

In order to make sense out of the number of cases, we must have a clear picture of the size and characteristics of the group of individuals in which the cases arose. A rate is useful only to the extent that the individual practitioner can decide to which kinds of patients the rate applies.

Ideally, the denominator of a rate would include all people who could have the condition or a representative sample of them. But what is relevant depends on one's perspective. For example, if we wanted to know the true prevalence of rheumatoid arthritis in Americans, we would prefer

Table 5.3
Ratio of the Prevalence of Conditions as Determined by Interview Divided by the Prevalence Determined by Physician Examination*

Hernia	1/5
Heart Condition	1/4
Peptic Ulcer	1/4
Diabetes	1/2.5
Hypertension	1/2
Arthritis	1/2
Asthma-Hay Fever	1.3/1
Chronic Bronchitis	1.5/1
Chronic Sinusitis	1.7/1

* From: Sanders BS. *Am J Publ Health*, 1962; 52:1648–1659.

to include in the denominator all people in the United States, rather than patients in office practice. But if one wanted to know the prevalence of rheumatoid arthritis in office practice—perhaps in order to plan services—the relevant denominator would be patients seen in office practice, not people in the population at large. In one survey, only 25% of adults found to have arthritic and rheumatic complaints (not necessarily rheumatoid arthritis) during a community survey had received services for such complaints from any health professional or institution (10).

Studying all individuals who might have or develop a given disease is rarely feasible. The next best alternative is to select a *representative sample* of all relevant individuals. A representative sample is a subgroup of the larger group, selected by a random procedure whereby every individual in the population has the same chance of being chosen for study. Only if the denominator group is selected in such a manner is it legitimate to generalize the findings of a study to all people in the population of interest.

Customarily, the group indicated in the denominator of a rate is referred to as the population or, more particularly the *population at risk*, where "at risk", means susceptible to the disease or outcome counted in the numerator. For example, it is not meaningful to describe the incidence or prevalence of cervical cancer in a population which includes women who have had hysterectomies, or includes men.

It is customary for epidemiologists to think of a population as consisting of all individuals residing in a geographic area. But as pointed out, in

Table 5.4

Rheumatoid Arthritis Diagnostic Criteria (American Rheumatism Association 1958 Revision)*

1. Morning stiffness.
2. Pain on motion or tenderness in at least one joint.†
3. Swelling (soft tissue thickening or fluid, not bony overgrowth alone) in at least one joint.†
4. Swelling of at least one other joint.†
5. Symmetrical joint swelling with simultaneous involvement of the same joint on both sides of the body.† Terminal phalangeal joint involvement will not satisfy the criterion.
6. Subcutaneous nodules over bony prominences, on extensor surfaces, or in juxta-articular regions.†
7. Roentgenographic changes typical of rheumatoid arthritis (which must include at least bony decalcification localized to or greatest around the involved joints and not just degenerative changes).
8. Positive agglutination (anti-gammaglobulin) test.
9. Poor mucin precipitate from synovial fluid (with shreds and cloudy solution).
10. Characteristic histologic changes in synovial membrane.
11. Characteristic histologic changes in nodules.

Categories	Number of Criteria Required	Minimum Duration of Continuous Symptoms
Classic	7 of 11	6 weeks (Nos. 1–5)
Definite	5 of 11	6 weeks (Nos. 1–5)
Probable	3 of 11	6 weeks (1 of Nos. 1–5)

* Adapted from: Ropes MW, Bennett CA, Cobb S, Jacox R, Jessar RA. 1958 revision of diagnostic criteria for rheumatoid arthritis. *Bull Rheum Dis*, 1958; 9:175–176.

† Observed by physician.

studies of clinical questions, the relevant populations generally consist of patients suffering from certain diseases or exhibiting certain clinical findings, and who are found in clinical settings which are similar to those in which the information will be used. Commonly, however, such patients are assembled at a limited number of clinical facilities where academic physicians see patients. In these instances, the population includes all patients with the appropriate findings from the hospitals or clinics involved. They may be a small and peculiar subset of all patients with the findings in some geographic area, as well as in office practice in general.

What difference might the choice of a population make? As discussed in Chapter 1, the incidence of further seizures in children who have had one febrile seizure varied from about 5% in the general population to as high as 75% in some clinics. Knowing which incidence is appropriate to one's patients is critical because it will influence the decision whether to begin chronic anticonvulsant treatment. The appropriate incidence depends upon the location and nature of the reader's practice. What is at issue is the generalizability of rates (Chapter 1). If the reader is an academic pediatric neurologist, referral center experience is more relevant. If the reader is a family physician or pediatrician providing community-based primary care, referral center experience may be irrelevant. Some of the authors reporting high incidences of subsequent seizures in children seen in referral centers argued that their high rate indicated that all such children should receive long-term anticonvulsant treatment. Such a conclusion may not be justified for the clinician in primary care practice, where the incidence of subsequent seizures is less than 5%.

THE USES OF INCIDENCE AND PREVALENCE

What purposes do incidence and prevalence serve? Practitioners use them in three different ways: predicting the future, describing things as they are, and making comparisons.

Predicting the Future

Incidence lends itself to estimating risk and predicting the future course of disease. Because incidence includes all cases occurring over time in a given group who initially were free from the outcome, it provides direct and relevant information about the probability of the outcome which can be used to predict for similar individuals (see Chapters 6 and 7). For incidence, the sequence of events is clear because the population was known to be free of the outcome at the outset and all cases were assessed.

On the other hand, prevalence describes the situation among a group of individuals at a given point in time; it offers no sound basis for predicting the future. If 30% of patients with stroke are depressed, this does not mean that 30% of stroke patients who are not currently depressed will become so in the future. It may be that depression predisposes to stroke or that non-depressed stroke patients are more likely to recover quickly. Because of the way in which they are measured, prevalences often reveal little about the sequence of events and only include a fraction of all possible cases. Thus, they are treacherous grounds for predicting the future.

The Probability that a Patient Has the Condition

Prevalence is particularly useful in guiding decisions about whether or not to use a diagnostic test as pointed out in Chapters 3 and 4, because prevalence is a determinant of predictive value. Knowing that a patient with a combination of demographic and clinical characteristics has a given probability of having the disease not only influences the interpretation of a diagnostic test result, but also may influence powerfully the selection among various treatment options.

The patient with pharyngitis, presented at the beginning of this chapter, illustrates how variations in prevalence can influence the approach to a clinical problem.

Example—Three approaches to the treatment of pharyngitis were compared. Their value was judged by weighing the potential benefits of preventing rheumatic fever with the costs of penicillin allergy. The three options included: obtain a throat culture and treat only those patients with throat cultures positive for β-hemolytic Group A streptococci; treat all patients without obtaining a culture; and neither culture nor treat any patient.

The analysis revealed that the optimal strategy depended upon the likelihood that a patient would have a positive culture, which can be estimated from the prevalence of streptococcal infection in the community at the time and the presence or absence of clinical findings such as fever. It was concluded that if the probability of a positive culture for an individual patient exceeds 20%, the patient should be treated; if it is less than 5%, the patient should not be cultured or treated; and if the probability lies between 5% and 20%, the patient should be cultured first and treatment based on the result (11).

Although the assumptions and computations involved in this analysis are complex, it represents a rational approach to the use of prevalences as indicators of individual probabilities of disease in guiding clinical decision-making.

Making Comparisons

Although isolated incidences and prevalences serve useful functions, as described previously, they become much more powerful tools in support of clinical decisions when used to make comparisons. It is the comparison between the frequencies of disease among individuals exposed to a factor, and individuals not exposed to the factor, that provides the best evidence suggesting causality, not just the commonness of the disease among those exposed. For example, the risk (incidence) of lung cancer among males who smoke heavily is of the order of 0.17% per year, hardly a common event. Only when this incidence is contrasted with the incidence in non-smokers (approximately 0.007% per year) does the devastating effect of smoking emerge. Clinicians use measures of frequency as the ingredients in comparative measures of the association between a factor and the disease or disease outcome. Ways of comparing rates will be described in more detail in Chapter 6.

SUMMARY

Most clinical questions are answered by reference to the commonness of events under varying circumstances. The commonness of clinical events is indicated by proportions or fractions whose numerators include the number of cases and whose denominators include the number of people from whom the cases arose.

The clinical reader will encounter two measures of commonness—incidence and prevalence. Incidence is the proportion of a susceptible group which develops new cases of the disease over an interval of time. Prevalence is the proportion of a group who have the disease at a single point in time.

Prevalence is measured by a single survey of a group containing cases and non-cases, while measurement of incidence requires examinations of a previously disease-free group over time. Thus, prevalence studies identify only those cases who are alive and diagnosable at the time of the survey whereas cohort (incidence) studies ascertain all new cases. Prevalent cases, therefore, may be a biased subset of all cases because they do not include those who have already succumbed or been cured. Additionally, prevalence studies frequently do not permit a clear understanding of the temporal relationship between a causal factor and a disease.

To make sense of incidence and prevalence, the clinician must understand the basis upon which the disease is diagnosed and the characteristics of the population represented in the denominator. The latter is of particular importance in trying to decide if a given measure of incidence or prevalence pertains to patients in one's own practice.

Incidence is the most appropriate measure of commonness with which to predict the future. Prevalence serves to quantitate the likelihood that a patient with certain characteristics has the disease at a single point in time, and is used for decisions about diagnosis and screening. The most powerful use of incidence and prevalence, however, is to compare different clinical alternatives.

POSTSCRIPT

Counting clinical events as described in this chapter may seem to be the most mundane of tasks. It seems so obvious that examining counts of clinical events under various circumstances is the foundation of clinical science. It may be worth reminding the reader that Pierre Louis introduced the "numerical method" of evaluating therapy less than 200 years ago. Dr. Louis had the audacity to count deaths and recoveries from febrile illness in the presence and absence of blood-letting. He was excoriated for allowing lifeless numbers to cast doubt on the healing powers of the leech, powers which had been amply confirmed by decades of astute qualitative clinical observation.

Suggested Reading

Ellenberg, JH, Nelson KB. Sample selection and the natural history of disease. *JAMA*, 1980; 243:1337–1340.

Friedman GD. Medical usage and abusage, "prevalence" and "incidence." *Ann Int Med* 1977; 84:502–504.

Morgenstern H, Kleinbaum DG, Kupper LL. Measures of disease incidence used in epidemiologic research. *Int J Epid* 1980; 9:97–104.

References

1. Friedman GD. Medical usage and abusage, "prevalence" and "incidence." *Ann Int Med*, 1977; 84:502–504.
2. Lowe TL, Tanaka K, Seashore MR, Young JG, Cohen DJ. Detection of phenylketonuria in autistic and psychotic children. *JAMA*, 1980; 243:126–128.
3. Yelin E, Meenan R, Nevitt M, Epstein W. Work disability in rheumatoid arthritis: effects of disease, social, and work factors. *Ann Int Med*, 1980; 93:551–556.
4. Asmundsson T, Kitburn KH. Survival after acute respiratory failure. *Ann Intern Med*, 1974; 80:54–57.
5. Sedlack RE, Whisnant J, Elveback LR, Kurland LT. Incidence of Crohn's disease in Olmsted County, Minnesota, 1935–1975. *Am J Epid*, 1980; 112:759–763.
6. Hulka BS, Redmond CK: Factors related to progression of cervical atypias. *Am J Epid*, 1971; 93:23–32.
7. Sanders BS. Have morbidity surveys been oversold? *Am J Publ Health* 1962; 52:1631–1637.
8. Rose CA: Chest pain questionnaire. *In*: Comparability in International Epidemiology. Acheson RM (Ed). New York: Milbank Memorial Fund, 1965; pages 32–40.
9. Ropes MW, Bennett GA, Cobb S, Jacox R, Jessar RA. 1958 revision of diagnostic criteria for rheumatoid arthritis. JJ Bunim (Ed). *Bull Rheum Dis*, 1958; 9:175–176.
10. Spitzer WO, Harth M, Goldsmith CH, Norman GR, et al. The arthritic complaint in primary care: prevalence, related disability, and costs. *J Rheum*, 1976; 3:88–99.
11. Tompkins RK, Burnes DC, Cable WE. An analysis of the cost-effectiveness of pharyngitis management and acute rheumatic fever prevention. *Ann Int Med*, 1977; 86:481–492.

chapter

6

Risk

Risk generally refers to the probability of some untoward event. In this chapter, the term risk is used in a more restricted sense to describe the likelihood that people who are without a disease, but exposed to certain factors ("risk factors"), will acquire the disease.

Members of our society have a strong interest in risk. Their concern has spawned popular books like Take Care of Yourself, Diet for Life, and The Healthy Heart. It is also reflected in headlines about the consequences of agent orange, nuclear accidents, birth control pills, and unnecessary surgery.

Often, questions about risk are taken to clinicians. Of course, people have their own ways of determining risk as well. Not everyone values the scientific method. "My grandfather smoked more than I do," a patient says, "and he lived to be 100!" But by and large, people value a scientific prediction of risk, and want expert advice.

In this chapter, we will consider how estimates of risk are obtained by observing the relationship between exposure to possible risk factors and the subsequent incidence of disease. Then we will describe several ways of comparing risks, both as they affect individuals and populations.

RISK FACTORS

Factors which are associated with an increased risk of acquiring disease are called *risk factors*. They cover a range of possibilities. Some are found in the physical environment, like toxins, infectious agents, and drugs. Some are part of the social environment. For example, disruption of family (e.g., loss of a spouse), daily routines, and culture have all been shown to increase rates of disease—not only emotional but physical illness as well. Other risk factors are behavioral, among them smoking, inactivity, and driving without seat belts. Risk factors are also inherited.

For example, having hemoglobin S increases risk for infection, particularly salmonella osteomyelitis.

Exposure to a risk factor means that a person has, before becoming ill, come in contact with or has manifested the factor in question. Exposure can take place at a point in time, as when someone comes in contact with an infectious disease or receives a drug, or may also be ongoing, like the risk of smoking for lung cancer or hypertension for stroke.

INFORMATION ABOUT RISK

Large and dramatic risks are easy for anyone to appreciate. Thus, it is not difficult to recognize the relationship between exposure and disease for conditions like chickenpox, sunburn, or asprin overdose because they follow exposure in a relatively rapid, certain, and obvious way. But much of the morbidity and mortality in our society is caused by chronic diseases. For these, the relationships between exposure and disease are far less obvious. It becomes virtually impossible for individual clinicians, however astute, to develop estimates of risk based on their own experiences with patients. This is true for several reasons, which are discussed below and summarized in Table 6.1.

Long Latency

Many chronic diseases have long latency periods between exposure to risk factors and the first manifestations of disease. Patients exposed during one time in a clinician's professional life may experience the consequences in another, years later, when the original exposure is all but forgotten. The link between exposure and disease is thereby obscured.

Frequent Exposure to Risk Factors

Many risk factors—such as cigarette smoking or driving when intoxicated—occur so frequently in our society that they scarcely seem dangerous. Only by looking at patterns of disease in large populations, or investigating special subgroups within it (e.g., Mormons who neither smoke nor drink), can we recognize risks which are in fact rather large.

Low Incidence of Disease

Most diseases, even ones thought to be "common", are actually quite rare. Thus, although lung cancer is the most common kind of cancer in men, the yearly incidence of lung cancer even in heavy smokers is less than 2/1,000. In the average physician's practice, then, years may pass between new cases of lung cancer. It is difficult to draw conclusions from such rare events.

Small Risk

If a factor confers only a small risk, a large number of "cases" are required to conclude that there is an association between the risk factor and disease. This is so even if both the risk factor and the disease occur relatively frequently. We are still struggling with whether cigarettes, coffee, and diabetes are risk factors for carcinoma of the pancreas, because estimates of risk are all small and, therefore, easily discounted as resulting from bias or chance. In contrast, it is not controversial that the human leukocyte antigen B-27 is a risk factor for spondylitis, because the antigen is present in most patients with spondylitis, and only a small proportion of people without the disease.

Common Disease

If the disease is one of those ordinarily occurring in our society—e.g., heart disease, cancer, or stroke—and some of the risk factors for it are already known, it becomes difficult to distinguish a new risk factor from the others. Also, there is less incentive to look for a new risk factor. For example, the syndrome of sudden and unexpected death is a fairly common way to die. Many cases seem related to coronary heart disease. However, it is entirely conceivable that there are other important causes,

Table 6.1
Conditions for which Personal Experience is Insufficient to Confirm Exposure-Risk Relationships

Long latency period between exposure and disease
Frequent exposure to risk factor
Low incidence of disease
Small risk from exposure
Common disease
Multiple causes of disease

as yet unrecognized because an adequate explanation for most cases is available.

On the other hand, rare diseases invite efforts to find a cause. Phocomelia is such an unusual congenital malformation that the appearance of just a few cases raised suspicion that some new agent (as it turned out, the drug, thalidomide) might be responsible. Similarly, physicians were quick to notice when several cases of carcinoma of the vagina, usually a very rare condition, began appearing. A careful search for an explanation was undertaken, and maternal exposure to diethylstilbesterol was found.

Multiple Causes

There is usually not a tight, one-to-one, relationship between a risk factor and one particular disease. Some people with hypertension develop congestive heart failure and many do not. Many people who do not have hypertension develop congestive heart failure as well. The relationship between hypertension and congestive heart failure is obscured by the fact that there are several other causes of the disease. Although people with hypertension are about three times more likely to develop congestive heart failure, and hypertension is the leading cause of that condition, physicians were not particularly attuned to this relationship until recently, when adequate data became available.

For these reasons, individual clinicians are rarely in a position to confirm associations between exposure and disease, though they may suspect them. For accurate information, they must turn to the medical literature, particularly studies which are carefully constructed and involve a large number of patients.

USES OF RISK

Information about risk serves several purposes.

Prediction

Risk is, of course, used to predict the future incidence of disease. How good that prediction is depends on the similarity of the patients upon whom the estimate of risk is based to the patients for whom the prediction is made. It has been shown that categories of risk for coronary heart disease derived from experience with a defined population (Framingham, Massachusetts) allow excellent predictions of the future incidence of coronary disease in the same population, and in similar populations (middle-aged white men and women in the continental United States) (1). The same categories distinguish between groups at relatively high and relatively low risk in very different populations, although the magnitude (incidence) of risk may be different. While risk for groups of people can be predicted rather well in this way, it is not possible to be precise about risk to any one individual in the group.

Diagnosis

The presence of a risk factor increases the probability that a disease is present. Knowledge of risk, therefore, can be used in the diagnostic process, inasmuch as increasing the prevalence of disease among patients tested is one way of improving the performance (positive predictive value) of a diagnostic test.

However, the presence of a risk factor usually increases the probability of disease very little for any one individual at one point in time, compared to other aspects of the clinical situation. For example, age and sex are relatively strong risk factors for coronary artery disease, yet the prevalence of disease in the most at-risk age and sex group, old men, is only 3.1% compared to 0.4% for the least at-risk group, young women. When specifics of the clinical situation—such as type of chest pain and results of an electrocardiographic stress test—are considered as well, the prevalence of coronary disease can be raised to 99.8% for old men, and 93.1% for young women (2).

More often, it is helpful to use the absence of a risk factor to help rule out disease, particularly when one factor is strong and predominant.

Thus, it would be reasonable to consider mesothelioma in the differential diagnosis of a pleural mass if the patient were an asbestos worker; but mesothelioma would be a long shot indeed if the patient had never been exposed to asbestos. Knowledge of risk factors is also used to improve the efficiency of screening programs by selecting subgroups of patients at increased risk.

Cause

It is often assumed that any excess incidence of disease in exposed over non-exposed persons is because one group was exposed. However, it is important to remember that risk factors need not be causes. A risk factor may mark a disease outcome indirectly, by virtue of its association with some other determinant(s) of disease—that is it may be confounded with a causal factor. This does not diminish the value of a risk factor as a way of predicting the risk of disease. But it does imply that removing such a risk factor might not remove the excess risk associated with it.

Prevention

If a risk factor is also a cause of disease, its removal can be used to prevent disease whether or not the mechanism by which the disease takes place is known. Some of the classics of epidemiology are illustrations. For example, before bacteria were identified Snow found an increased rate of cholera among people drinking water supplied by a particular company, and controlled an epidemic by cutting off that supply. The concept of cause and its relationship to prevention will be discussed in Chapter 11.

STUDIES OF RISK

There are several strategies for determining risk. In general, there is a trade-off between scientific rigor and feasibility.

Observational Studies

To a scientist, the most satisfactory way of determining whether exposure to a potential risk factor results in an increased risk of disease would be to conduct an experiment. Subjects currently without disease would be divided into groups of equal susceptibility to the disease in question. One group would be exposed to the purported risk factor and the other would not, but the groups would otherwise be treated the same. Later, any difference in observed rates of disease in the groups could be attributed to the risk factor.

Unfortunately, the effects of most risk factors cannot be studied in this way. Consider some of the questions of risk that concern us today. Does saccharin cause bladder cancer? Are inactive or obese people more subject to cardiovascular disease? Have the chemicals at Love Canal or the radioactivity at Three-Mile Island increased the risk of disease among local residents? For questions like these, exposure is not and cannot be determined as part of an experiment. Subjects become exposed or not for reasons that have nothing to do with the scientific value of the information their exposure may provide. As a result, it is usually necessary to study risk in less obtrusive ways.

Clinical studies in which the researcher gathers data by simply observing events as they happen, without playing an active part in what takes place, are called *observational studies*. They are contrasted with experimental studies in which the researcher determines who is exposed. Although experimental studies are more scientifically rigorous, observational studies are the only feasible way of studying most questions of risk.

Observational studies are feasible, but subject to a great many more potential biases than are experiments. When people become exposed or not exposed to a certain risk factor, in the natural course of events, they are also likely to differ in a great many other ways. If these are related to disease as well, they could account for any association observed between risk factors and disease.

This leads to the main challenge of observational studies: to deal with unwanted differences between exposure groups in order to mimic as closely as possible an experiment. The differences are considered "unwanted" from the point of view of someone trying to determine cause-effect relationships. The following example illustrates one approach.

Example—Although sickle-cell trait (HbAS) is generally regarded as a benign condition, several studies have suggested that it is associated with defects in physical growth and cognitive development. A study was undertaken, therefore, to see if children born with HbAS experienced problems in growth and development more frequently than children with normal hemoglobin (HbAA), everything else being equal. It was recognized that a great many other factors are related both to growth and development and also to having HbAS. Among these are: race, sex, birth date, birth weight, gestational age, five-minute Apgar score, and socioeconomic status. If these were not taken into account, it would not be possible to distinguish the effects of HbAS, in and of itself, from the effects of the other factors. The authors chose to deal with these other factors by matching. For each child with HbAS, they selected a child with HbAA who was similar with respect to the seven other factors. Fifty newborns with HbAS and 50 with HbAA were followed from birth to 3–5 years old. No differences in growth and development were found (3).

Other ways of dealing with differences between groups will be described in the next chapter (Chapter 7).

Cohorts

The term *cohort* is used to describe a group of people who have something in common when they are first assembled, and who are then observed for a period of time to see what happens to them. A cohort can have any of a number of things in common at first, depending on the question it is being used to answer. Table 6.2 lists some of the ways in which the concept of cohorts is used in clinical research.

Whatever members of a cohort have in common, observations of them should fulfill two criteria if they are to provide sound information.

First, cohorts should be observed over a meaningful period of time in the natural history of the disease in question. This is so that there will be sufficient time for the risk to be expressed. If we wish to learn whether neck irradiation during childhood results in thyroid neoplasms, a five-year follow-up would not be a fair test of the risk associated with irradiation, because the usual time period between exposure and the onset of this disease is considerably longer.

Second, all members of the cohort should all be observed over the full period of follow-up. To the extent that people drop out of the cohort, and their reasons for dropping out are related in some way to the outcome,

Table 6.2

Cohorts and their Purposes

Characteristic in Common	To Assess Effect of	Example
Age	Age	Life expectancy for people age 70 (regardless of when born)
Date of birth	Calendar time	Tuberculosis rates for people born in 1910
Exposure	Risk factor	Lung cancer in people who smoke
Disease	Prognosis	Survival rate for patients with breast cancer
Treatment	Intervention	Improvement in survival for patients with Hodgkin's disease given radiotherapy

the information provided by an incomplete cohort can be a distortion of the true state of affairs.

Cohort Studies

In a *cohort study*, a group of people (a cohort) is assembled, none of whom have experienced the outcome of interest. On entry to the study, people in the cohort are classified according to those characteristics that might be related to outcome. These people are then followed over time to see which of them experience the outcome. It is then possible to see how initial characteristics relate to subsequent outcome events. A cohort study is diagrammed in Figure 6.1. Other names for such studies are longitudinal (emphasizing that patients are followed over time), prospective (implying the forward direction in which the patients are pursued), and incidence (calling attention to the basic measure of disease events over time).

The following is a description of a classical cohort study, which has made an extremely important contribution to our understanding of cardiovascular disease.

Example—The Framingham Study was begun in 1949 to identify factors associated with an increased risk of coronary heart disease (CHD). A representative sample of 5209 men and women, aged 30–59, was selected from approximately 10,000 persons of that age living in Framingham, a small town near Boston. Of these, 5127 were free of CHD when first examined and, therefore, at risk of developing CHD subsequently. These people have been re-examined biennially for evidence of coronary disease. The study has run for 30 years, and has demonstrated that risk of developing CHD is associated with blood pressure, serum cholesterol, cigarette smoking, glucose intolerance and left ventricular hypertrophy. There is a large difference in risk between those with none and those with all of these risk factors (4).

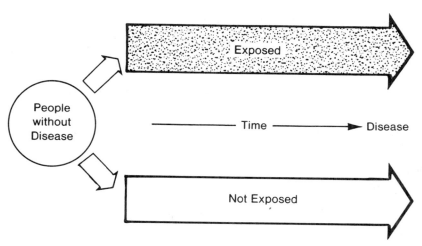

Figure 6.1.   Design of A Cohort Study of Risk.

Historical Cohort Studies

Cohort studies can be conducted in two ways (Figure 6.2). The cohort can be assembled in the present and followed into the future (a *concurrent cohort study*); or it can be identified from past records and followed forward from that time up to the present (an *historical cohort study*).

Most of the advantages and disadvantages of cohort studies, as strategies, apply whether they are concurrent or historical. However, the potential for difficulties with the quality of data is different for the two. In concurrent studies, data can be collected specifically for the purposes of the study, and with full anticipation of what is needed. It is thereby possible to avoid biases that might undermine the accuracy of the data. On the other hand, data for historical cohorts are often gathered for other purposes—usually as part of medical records for patient care. These data may not be of sufficient quality for rigorous research.

Survival Cohorts

In true cohort studies, whether historical or concurrent, patients are assembled at the beginning of the period of time during which they are observed and their course described as it unfolds from that point. True cohort studies should be distinguished from another kind of study in which a group of people with a condition is observed over time, but assembled at different points in the course of their disease. Sometimes patients are included in a study because they both have a disease and are currently available—perhaps because they are being seen in a specialized clinic. Their clinical course is then described by going back in time and seeing how they have fared up to the present. A *survival cohort* is the

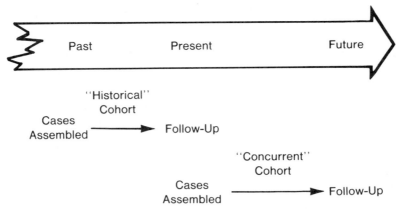

Figure 6.2. Historical and Concurrent Cohort Studies.

name given to a group of people who are assembled at various times in the course of their disease, rather than at the beginning.

Survival cohorts are often interpreted as if they were a description of the course of disease from its inception. However, they are usually a biased view of the course of disease because they include only those patients who have survived and are available for study sometime after their disease began. For lethal conditions, the patients are the ones who are fortunate enough to have survived and so are available for observation years later. For diseases which remit, the patients are the ones who are unfortunate enough to have persistent disease. The difference between true cohorts, identified at the beginning of follow-up, and cases found later in the course of disease, is illustrated in Chapter 5, Figure 5.3.

Reports of survival cohorts are misleading if they are presented as true cohorts. Survival cohorts are relatively prevalent in the medical literature, particularly in the form of "case reports" (to be discussed in Chapter 10).

Limitations of Cohort Studies

Cohort studies of risk are the best available substitute for a true experiment, when experimentation is not possible. However, they present a considerable number of practical difficulties of their own. Some of the advantages and disadvantages of cohort studies, for the purpose of describing risk factors, are summarized in Table 6.3. If the outcome they set out to observe is infrequent, and most are, a large number of subjects must be entered in a study and remain under surveillance for a long time before results are available. For example, the Framingham Study of coronary heart disease was the largest of its kind, and studied one of the most frequent of the chronic diseases in our society. Nevertheless, over 5000 people had to be followed for several years before the first prelimi-

Table 6.3

Advantages and Disadvantages of Cohort Studies

Advantages	Disadvantages
The only way of establishing incidence (i.e., absolute risk) directly	Inefficient, because many more subjects must be enrolled than experience the event of interest. Therefore: cannot be used for rare diseases
Follow the same logic as the clinical question: if persons exposed, then get the disease?	Expensive because of resources necessary to study many people over time
Exposure can be elicited without the bias that might occur if outcome were already known	Results not available for a long time
Can assess the relationship between exposure and many diseases	Can assess the effects of exposure to relatively few factors (i.e., those recorded at the outset.)

nary conclusions could be published. Only 5% of the people had experienced a coronary event during the first eight years!

Another problem with cohort studies results from the fact that the people being studied are usually "free-living" and not under the control of researchers. A great deal of effort and money must be expended to keep track of them. Cohort studies, therefore, are expensive, sometimes costing millions of dollars.

Because of the time and money required for cohort studies, this approach cannot be used for all clinical questions about risk. For practical reasons, the cohort approach has been reserved for only the most important questions. This has led to efforts to find more efficient, yet dependable, ways of assessing risk. One of these ways, case control studies, will be discussed in Chapter 10.

COMPARING RISKS

The basic expression of risk is incidence, defined in Chapter 5 as the number of new cases of disease arising in a defined population during a given period of time. But usually we want to compare the incidence of disease in two or more cohorts, which have different exposures to some possible risk factor. To compare risks, several measures of the association between exposure and disease, called "measures of effect", are commonly used. They represent different concepts of risk and are used for different

Table 6.4
Measures of effect

Expression	Question	Definition*
Attributable risk (Risk difference)	What is the incidence of disease attributable to exposure?	$AR = I_E - I_{\bar{E}}$
Relative risk (Risk ratio)	How many times more likely are exposed persons to become diseased, relative to non-exposed?	$RR = \dfrac{I_E}{I_{\bar{E}}}$
Population attributable risk	What is the incidence of disease in a population, associated with the occurrence of a risk factor?	$AR_P = AR \times P$
Population attributable fraction	What fraction of disease in a population is attributable to exposure to a risk factor?	$AF_P = \dfrac{AR_P}{R_T}$

* Where:
I_E = incidence in exposed persons
$I_{\bar{E}}$ = incidence in non-exposed persons
P = prevalence of exposure to a risk factor
R_T = total incidence of disease in a population

purposes. Four measures of effect are summarized in Table 6.4, and illustrated by an example in Table 6.5.

Attributable Risk

First, one might ask what is the additional risk (incidence) following exposure, over and above that experienced by people who are not exposed. The answer is expressed as *attributable risk*, the incidence of disease in exposed persons minus the incidence in non-exposed persons. Attributable risk is the additional incidence of disease related to exposure, taking into account the background incidence of disease, presumably from other causes, that would have occurred even among those not exposed. Because of the way it is calculated, attributable risk is also called "risk difference."

Relative Risk

On the other hand, one might ask, "how many times more likely are exposed persons to get the disease relative to non-exposed?" To answer this question, we speak of *relative risk* or risk ratio, the ratio of incidence in exposed persons to incidence in non-exposed persons. Relative risk tells us nothing about the magnitude of absolute risk (incidence). Even

Table 6.5
Calculating Measures of Effect. Cigarette Smoking and Death from Lung Cancer*

Simple Risks

Death rate from lung cancer in cigarette smokers	0.96/1000/year
Death rate from lung cancer in non-smokers	0.07/1000/year
Prevalence of cigarette smoking	56%
Total death rate from lung cancer	0.56/1000/year

Compared Risks

Attributable risk $= 0.96/1000/\text{year} - 0.07/1000/\text{year}$

$\qquad = 0.89/1000/\text{year}$

Relative risk $\quad = \dfrac{0.96/1000/\text{year}}{0.07/1000/\text{year}}$

$\qquad = 13.7$

Population attributable risk $= 0.89/1000/\text{year} \times 0.56$

$\qquad = 0.50/1000/\text{year}$

Population attributable fraction $= \dfrac{0.50/1000/\text{year}}{0.56/1000/\text{year}}$

$\qquad = 0.89$

* Estimated data from: Doll R, Hill AB. *Br Med J*, 1964; 1:1399–1410.

for large relative risks, the absolute risk might be quite small if the disease is uncommon. It does tell us the strength of the association between exposure and disease, and so is a useful measure of effect for studies of disease etiology.

Interpreting Risk

The clinical judgments attached to relative and attributable risk are often quite different, because the two stand for entirely different concepts. The appropriate expression of risk depends upon the question being asked.

Example—The Royal College of General Practitioners has been conducting a study of the health effects of oral contraceptives. During 1968 and 1969, over 23,000 women taking oral contraceptives, and an equal number of women who had never taken the pill, were entered into the study by 1400 physicians. These physicians subsequently reported oral contraceptive use, morbidity, and mortality twice a year. The use of oral contraceptives was updated regularly. After 10 years of follow-up, it was reported that oral contraceptive users had a risk of dying from circulatory diseases that was 4.2 times greater than for non-users. But the risk of dying was increased by only 22.7/100,000 women-years. An individual woman, weighing the risks of oral contraceptives, must deal with the two very different concepts of risk. On the one hand, a four-fold greater risk of dying might loom large. On the other, two chances in 10,000 is a very remote possibility (5).

In general, because attributable risk represents the actual probability of disease in those exposed, it is a more meaningful expression of risk in most clinical situations.

Population Risk

Another way of looking at risk is to ask: how much does a risk factor contribute to the overall rates of disease in groups of people, rather than individuals. This information would be useful for deciding which risk factors are particularly important, and which trivial, to the overall health of a community, and so it could inform those in policy positions how to choose priorities for the deployment of health care resources.

To estimate population risk, it is necessary to take into account the frequency with which members of a community are exposed to a risk factor (6). A relatively weak risk factor which is quite prevalent could contribute more to overall risk in a community than a stronger risk factor which is rarely present.

Population attributable risk is a measure of the excess incidence of disease in a community that is associated with the occurrence of a risk factor. It is the product of the attributable risk and the prevalence of the risk factor in a population.

One can also express the fraction of disease occurrence in a population which is associated with a particular risk factor, called the *population attributable fraction*. It is defined as the population attributable risk divided by the total incidence of disease in the population.

Figure 6.3 illustrates how the prevalence of a risk factor determines the relationship between individual and population risk. *A* shows the attributable risk of death according to diastolic blood pressure. Risk increases with increasing blood pressure. However, few people have extremely high blood pressure (*B*). When "hypertension" is taken to be a diastolic blood pressure $\geq$ 90 mm Hg, most hypertensive people are just over 90 and very few are in the highest category, 110–120 mm Hg. As a result (*C*), the greatest percentage of excess deaths in the population (58.4%) is attributable to relatively low-grade hypertension, 90–105 mm Hg. Paradoxically, then, physicians could save more lives by effective treatment of mild hypertension than severe hypertension.

Measures of population risk are less frequently encountered in the clinical literature than are measures of individual risk (e.g., attributable and relative risk). But a particular practice is as much a population for its health care providers as is a community for health policy-makers. Also, the concept of how the prevalence of exposure affects risk in groups

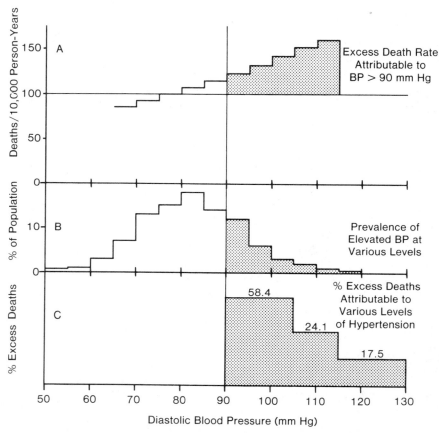

Figure 6.3. Relationships Among Attributable Risk, Prevalence of Risk Factor, and Population Risk for Hypertension. (Adapted from: The Hypertension Detection and Follow-up Cooperative Group. *Ann NY Acad Sci*, 1978; 304:254–266.)

can be important in the care of individual patients. For instance, when patients cannot give a history, or when exposure is difficult for them to recognize, we depend on the usual prevalence of exposure to estimate the likelihood of various diseases. When considering treatable causes of cirrhosis in a North American patient, for example, it would be more profitable to consider alcohol than schistosomes, inasmuch as few North

Americans are exposed to schistosoma mansoni. Of course, one might take a very different stance in the Nile Delta, where people rarely drink alcohol and schistosomes are prevalent.

SUMMARY

Risk factors are characteristics which are associated with an increased risk of becoming diseased. Whether or not a particular risk factor is a cause of disease, its presence allows one to predict the probability that disease will occur.

Most suspected risk factors cannot be manipulated for the purposes of an experiment, so it is usually necessary to study risk by simply observing people's experience with risk factors and disease. One way of doing so is to select a cohort of people who are and are not exposed to a risk factor, and observe their subsequent incidence of disease.

When disease rates are compared, the results can be expressed in several ways. Attributable risk is the excess incidence of disease related to exposure. Relative risk is the number of times more likely exposed people are to become diseased, relative to non-exposed. The impact of a risk factor on groups of people takes into account not only the risk related to exposure, but the prevalence of exposure as well.

Although it is scientifically preferable to study risk by means of cohort studies, this approach is not always feasible because of the time, effort and expense they entail.

Suggested Reading

Dawber TR. The Framingham Study. The Epidemiology of Atherosclerotic Disease. Cambridge, Massachusetts: Harvard U. Press, 1980.

Feinstein AR. Clinical Biostatistics. Section 1. The Architecture of Cohort Research. St. Louis: C. V. Mosby, Co., 1977.

Gordon T, Kannel WB, Halperin M. Predictability of coronary heart disease. *J Chron Dis,* 1979; 32:427–440.

Lilienfeld AM. Foundations of Epidemiology. Chapter 9. Prospective Studies. New York: Oxford University Press, 1976.

References

1. Gordon T, Kannel WB, Halperin M. Predictability of coronary heart disease. *J Chron Dis,* 1979; 32:427–440.
2. Diamond GA, Forrester JS. Analysis of probability as an aid in the clinical diagnosis of coronary-artery disease. *N Engl J Med,* 1979; 300:1350–1358.
3. Kramer MS, Rooks Y, Pearson HA. Growth and development in children with sickle-cell trait. *N Engl J Med,* 1978; 299:686–689.
4. Dawber TR. The Framingham Study. The Epidemiology of Atherosclerotic Disease. Cambridge, Massachusetts. Harvard University Press, 1980.
5. Royal College of General Practitioners' Oral Contraception Study. Further analysis of mortality in oral contraceptive users. *Lancet,* 1981; 1:541–546.
6. Deubner DC, Tyroler HA, Cassel JC, Hames CG, Becker C. Attributable risk, population attributable risk, and population attributable fraction of death associated with hypertension in a biracial population. *Circulation,* 1975; 52:901–908.

chapter

7

Prognosis

When people become sick, they have a great many questions about how their illness will affect them. Is it dangerous? Could I die of it? Will there be pain? How long will I be able to continue my present activities? Will it ever go away altogether? Most patients want to know what to expect, whether or not anything can be done about their illness.

Prognosis is a prediction of the future course of disease following its onset. In this chapter, we will deal with the various ways in which the course of disease can be estimated and expressed. Our intention is to give readers a better understanding of a difficult but indispensible task: predicting patients' futures as closely as possible. The object is to avoid expressing prognosis with vagueness when it is unnecessary, and with certainty when it is misleading.

PROBABILITY AND THE INDIVIDUAL

Prognosis is expressed as the probability that something will occur in the future. We summarize past experience with patients, for example, as an incidence of events, and use that to predict what will occur, on the average, among similar patients. If our knowledge of human disease were more complete, and if disease behaved in a more predictable manner, we would not need to resort to probability. But we do not have that luxury.

There is a basic mismatch between probability and the individual. Quite naturally, both patients and physicians would like to answer questions about the future course of disease as precisely as possible. They are uncomfortable assigning a probability, like the probability of living five years, to an individual. Moreover, any one patient will, at the end of five years, have either lived or died. So, in a sense, the average is always wrong for the individual, because it is expressed in different terms. The prediction is a probability, usually falling between zero and one, whereas the actual event, when it occurs, is described by a probability of either zero or one.

Nevertheless, knowledge of prognosis does help us to select a management strategy. Even if a prediction does not come true in an individual case, it will usually be borne out with many such cases. After all, weather forecasts are not always accurate either, but they do help us decide whether to carry an umbrella.

DIFFERENCE BETWEEN RISK AND PROGNOSIS

Although risk and prognosis have many similarities, and both are assessed by means of cohort studies, a distinction should be made between conditions which increase the risk of getting a disease and those which predict the course once the disease is present. The former, as discussed in Chapter 6, are called risk factors: conditions that can be identified in well persons and, when present, are associated with an increased risk of acquiring disease. The latter are called *prognostic factors*: conditions which, when present in persons already known to have disease, are associated with an outcome of the disease.

The difference between risk and prognosis is illustrated in Figure 7.1 for acute myocardial infarction. A somewhat arbitrary distinction is made between events that occur before and after the disease has been recognized.

If risk and prognosis fall along the same continuum in the course of disease, why consider them separately? We touched on this question in the preceding chapter, and will elaborate here.

Difference in Rates

First, risk factors generally predict low-probability events. Yearly rates for the onset of various diseases are in the order of 1/100 to 1/10,000. As a result, relationships between exposure and risk usually elude even astute clinicians unless they rely on carefully executed studies, often involving a large number of subjects over an extended period of time. Prognosis, on the other hand, describes relatively frequent events. Clinicians can form some sort of estimate of prognosis on their own, from their personal experience. Of course, these estimates can be made more precise by rigorous methods.

Nature of Events

Risk and prognosis usually are described in different terms. For risk, the event being counted is the onset of disease. For prognosis, a variety of consequences of disease are counted, including death, complications, disability, suffering, etc. These events will be considered later in this chapter.

Differences in Factors

Risk factors and prognostic factors are not necessarily the same. They are often considerably different for a given disease. For example, low blood pressure decreases one's chances of having an acute myocardial infarction, but is a bad prognostic sign when present during an acute event (Figure 7.1). Similarly, exogenous estrogens during menopause increase women's risk of endometrial cancer, but the associated cancers are found at an earlier stage, and so seem to have a better than average prognosis.

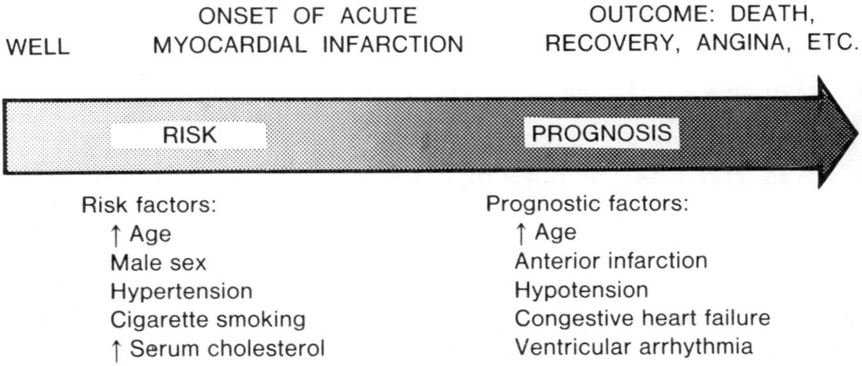

	ONSET OF ACUTE	OUTCOME: DEATH,
WELL	MYOCARDIAL INFARCTION	RECOVERY, ANGINA, ETC.

RISK   PROGNOSIS

Risk factors:
 ↑ Age
 Male sex
 Hypertension
 Cigarette smoking
 ↑ Serum cholesterol

Prognostic factors:
 ↑ Age
 Anterior infarction
 Hypotension
 Congestive heart failure
 Ventricular arrhythmia

Figure 7.1. Difference between Risk and Prognosis for Acute Myocardial Infarction.

Some factors do have a similar effect on both risk and prognosis. Men are more likely than women to acquire coronary disease in middle age, and are also more likely to die if they get it. Also, both the risk of experiencing an acute myocardial infarction, and the risk of dying of it increase with age.

NATURAL HISTORY/CLINICAL COURSE

Natural History

Clinicians often want to know the *natural history* of disease. "Natural" implies that they want to know the evolution of disease without medical intervention; that is, how patients will fare if nothing is done for their disease.

Is it practical even to ask this question in countries where medical care is so sought after and available? That depends on the disease. A great many diseases generally do not come under medical care during a large part of their course, if at all. They remain unrecognized, perhaps because they are asymptomatic or are considered among the ordinary discomforts of daily living. Mild depression, anemia, and cancers which are occult and slow growing (e.g., some cancers of the thyroid and prostate) are examples of such diseases.

Clinical Course

There are other diseases for which patients regularly come under medical care at some time in the course of their illness. These diseases tend to assume a high profile because they result in symptoms like pain, failure to thrive, disfigurement, or unusual behavior which compel patients or their families to seek care. Examples include juvenile diabetes mellitis, carcinoma of the lung, and rabies. Once disease is recognized, it is also likely to be treated. The term *clinical course* has been used to describe the evolution of disease which has come under medical care, and is then treated in a variety of ways which might affect the subsequent course of events.

Sampling Bias

Descriptions of the course of disease are based on samples, and so are susceptible to a sampling bias.

Published accounts of disease which are based on experience in special centers can paint a misleading picture of the disease in less selected patients. The recognized cases may be particularly symptomatic, or may have come to attention because the patients had other symptoms which are not related to the disease. Therefore, it is important to ask just how natural the history we observe is. The true natural history of unselected cases of a disease, and the course of those that are recognized, can be quite different.

Example—Hereditary Spherocytosis (HS) is a defect of red cell membranes which is inherited as an autosomal dominant. In its classical form, HS is characterized by hemolytic anemia, splenomegaly, and the presence of spherical red cells which can be seen on blood smears. Usually production of red cells keeps pace with hemolysis; but anemia can be severe if production is reduced for some reason, like acute infection or old age. A definitive diagnosis can be made by testing red cells for osmotic fragility.

Although some people with HS are severely affected, a great many others are asymptomatic. Having no reasons to consult physicians, or to have special tests done, they generally escape detection and so contribute little to our picture of the usual course of HS. This should be borne in mind when counselling patients who are well and are discovered to have HS only because they were screened, after a relative was found to have the disease.

Even for diseases that regularly come under care, prognoses reported in the medical literature may be systematically different from the usual course of disease, as pointed out in Chapter 1. Most academic physicians' experience, and most published reports, come from medical centers; and patients seen in medical centers are usually not a representative sample of patients who are in the community and cared for by local physicians. In fact, the reasons for referral are often related to prognosis. Many patients are sent because they are doing badly. Perhaps the usual treatments have been given and have not worked. Sometimes the patient has an unusual or perplexing complication of disease, or other features which suggest trouble is brewing. Under these circumstances, it is natural for both patients and physicians to seek more expert opinion.

The following is an example of how sampling bias can affect our understanding of prognosis.

Example—Multiple Sclerosis (MS) seems to be a crippling and lethal disease when seen from the perspective of neurology clinics and hospitals. However, when the clinical course of MS is described for all patients developing the disease in a defined geographic region, a different picture emerges. In one such study (Figure 7.2) one-half of the patients were alive 50 years after onset, about the same number as would have been expected for people of the same age and sex who did not have MS. Most patients were alive and ambulatory 10 years after diagnosis (1).

As a general rule, reports of prognosis based on experience in medical centers cannot be taken as an accurate guide to prognosis in less selected medical settings. Usually reported cases will have a worse than average prognosis.

OUTCOMES OF DISEASE

Descriptions of prognosis should include the full range of manifestations that would be considered important to patients. By this is meant not only death and disease, but also conditions like pain, anguish, and inability to care for one's self or pursue usual activities.

In their efforts to be "scientific," physicians sometimes value certain kinds of outcomes over others, at the expense of clinical relevance. Clinical events which cannot be directly perceived by patients—for example, reduction in tumor size, normalization of blood chemistries, or change in serology—are not ends in themselves. They can serve as proxies for suffering and death if it is known that they are good proxies. Thus, hypercalcemia is an important clinical outcome of hyperparathyroidism only if it causes symptoms like drowsiness or thirst or if there is reason to believe that it will eventually lead to complications like bone or kidney disease. If an outcome cannot be related to something patients will recognize, the information cannot be used to guide patient care, although it may be of considerable value in understanding the origins and mechanisms of disease.

When describing prognosis, data should be included because of their importance in the clinical situation and not because they can be measured precisely or are measured in a particular way. A patient recently seen by one of us illustrates the problem.

Example—A 50-year old man was admitted to the coronary care unit with an acute myocardial infarction. By the second day, he was "clinically" well with no signs of congestive heart failure, pain, or arrhythmia. However, his serum creatine

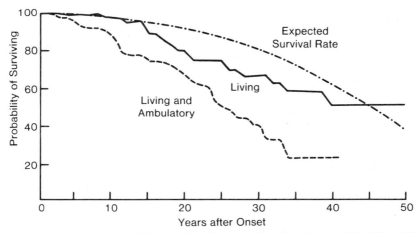

Figure 7.2. Prognosis of Disease in a Community. Survival and Mobility After the Onset of Multiple Sclerosis (Redrawn from: Percy AK, Nobrega FT, Okazaki H, Glattre E, Kurland LT. *Arch Neurol*, 1971; 25:105–111.)

phosphokinase (CPK) had risen to extremely high levels, over 2000 units/ml. Some of his physicians, citing evidence that high CPK levels are associated with a poor prognosis, believed he had a massive myocardial infarction, and argued that his prognosis was, therefore, so dismal that he should not be resuscitated if he suffered a cardiac arrest. Others considered the absence of complications evidence for a mild myocardial infarction, consistent with an excellent recovery. The patient did, in fact, have an uneventful clinical course, despite his very alarming laboratory test result.

Table 7.1 provides a view of how outcomes are described to physicians in the general medical literature. It is apparent that authors of research articles are particularly fond of "hard," biologic data, of the sort provided by diagnostic tests. On the other hand, outcomes of even greater importance to patients such as the ability to carry on daily activities receive short shrift, even in reports of prognosis or the effects of treatment, where such outcomes are clinically important. At best, the medical literature does not provide much information about some important outcomes of disease. At worst, it may change the reader's perceptions about what is important in clinical medicine.

PROGNOSIS AS A RATE

It is convenient to summarize the course of disease as a single number. Rates commonly used for this purpose are shown in Table 7.2. These rates have in common the same basic components of incidence: events arising in a cohort of patients over time (Chapter 5). However, some of the components of the rates are not made explicit, and this must be borne in mind when interpreting the rate.

Table 7.1

Outcomes of Disease Reported in the Medical Literature*

Outcome	% of Articles
Diagnostic Tests	90
Physical Signs	68
Symptoms	63
Death	18
Social or Occupational Function	3
Mental Status	1

* For *N Engl J Med*, *JAMA*, and *Lancet*, 1976. From: Fletcher RH, Fletcher SW. *N Engl J Med* 1979; 301:180–183.

Assumptions

First, the interval of follow-up is not specified for several of the rates. The interval is taken to be an adequate period of time for all the events to occur, but that is not always the case. Any period of follow-up which falls short will lower observed rates, relative to the true ones.

Second, for rates involving death, it is generally assumed that there are no important causes of death other than the disease in question. If there are, the effect of these deaths on reported survival rates will depend on how they are handled. Deaths included with the rest will decrease apparent survival from the disease. But, if these patients are removed from the study, survival rates will seem more favorable because fewer patients will be at risk of dying from the disease being considered.

Third, all rates must begin at some point in the course of disease such as onset of symptoms, diagnosis, or treatment. Quite naturally, rates are heavily influenced by the way in which "zero-time" is assigned.

Example—In a study of the value of detecting breast cancer by routine mammography and breast examination, it was found that women whose cancers were detected by these special means had a lower death rate than those whose cancers were found in the ordinary course of events. The investigators were concerned that the difference might have resulted from assigning the "onset" of breast cancer earlier for the screened women, so that an improvement in survival would have been found whether or not subsequent treatment were more effective. A correction was made for this difference in zero-time, and the improvement in survival persisted, confirming the value of screening (and earlier treatment) for breast cancer (2).

A Tradeoff: Simplicity versus Loss of Information

Expressing prognosis as a rate has the virtue of simplicity. Rates can be committed to memory and communicated succinctly. Their drawback

Table 7.2
Rates Commonly Used to Describe Prognosis

Rate	Definition
Five-year Survival	Percent of patients surviving five years from some point in the course of their disease
Case-Fatality	Percent of patients with a disease who die of it.*
Response	Percent of patients showing some evidence of improvement following an intervention*
Remission	Percent of patients entering a phase in which disease is no longer detectable.*
Recurrence	Percent of patients who have return of disease after a disease-free interval.*

* Time under observation is either stated, or assumed to be sufficiently long so that all events that will occur have been observed.

is that very little information is conveyed, so that vast differences in prognosis can be hidden within similar summary rates.

Figure 7.3 shows five-year survival for patients with four conditions. For each condition, about 10% of the patients are alive at five years. But the crude 10% fails to express differences of considerable importance. In *A*, patients with lung cancer presenting as a solitary pulmonary nodule die more rapidly at first than they do later, suggesting that the tumors are responsible for early death, after which the risk associated with the tumor falls off. *B* shows that patients with dissecting aneurysm experience a huge mortality early on; but if they survive the first few months, their risk of dying is not affected by having had the dissection. Chronic myelocytic leukemia (*C*) is a condition which has relatively little effect on survival during the first few years after diagnosis. Later, there is an acceleration in mortality rate until nearly all patients are dead five years after diagnosis. *D* is presented as a bench mark. Only at age 100 do people in the general population have a five-year survival rate comparable to that of patients with the three diseases.

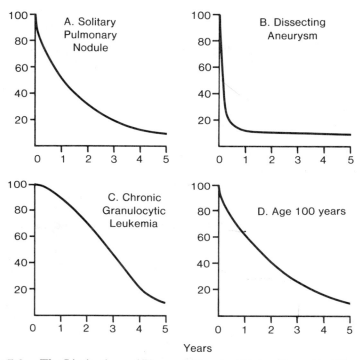

Figure 7.3. The Limitations of Five-year Survival Rates. Four Conditions With the Same Five-year Survival of 10%. (Data from: Steele JD. The Solitary Pulmonary Nodule. Springfield, IL. Charles C Thomas, 1964; Anagnostopoulos CE, Manakavalan JS, Prabhaker MD, Kittle CF. *Am J Cardiol,* 1972; 30:263–273; Kardinal CG, Bateman JR, Weiner J. *Arch Intern Med,* 1976; 136:305–313; 1979 Life Insurance Fact Book. Washington, American College of Life Insurance, 1979.)

SURVIVAL ANALYSIS

When interpreting prognosis, we would like to know the likelihood, on the average, that patients with a given condition will experience an outcome at any point in time. When prognosis is expressed as a summary rate it does not contain this information. However, a method called *survival analysis* results in information about average time-to-event for any time in the course of disease.

Survival of a Cohort

The most straightforward way to learn about survival is to assemble a cohort of patients with the condition at some point in the course of their illness (e.g., onset of symptoms, diagnosis, or beginning of treatment) and keep them under observation until all have experienced the outcome of interest. One might then represent the experience with these patients'. course of disease as shown in Figure 7.4. The plot of survival against time

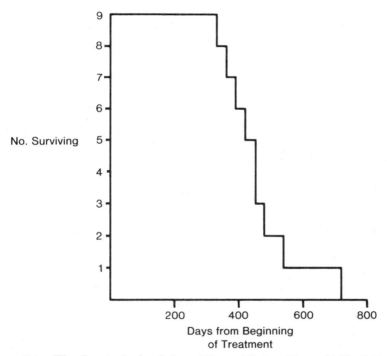

Figure 7.4. The Survival of a Cohort Where All Are Observed Until Death. Nine Patients with Glioblastoma Multiforme Treated with BCNU. (Data from: Rudnick S. Unpublished.)

displays steps, corresponding to the death of each of the nine patients in the cohort. If the number of patients were increased, the size of the steps would diminish; if a very large number of patients were represented, the figure would approximate a smooth curve. This information could then be used to predict the year by year, or even week by week, prognosis of similar patients.

Unfortunately, getting the information in this way would be quite inefficient for several reasons. Some of the patients would undoubtedly drop out of the study before the end of the follow-up period, perhaps because of another illness, a move to a place where follow-up was impractical or because of dissatisfaction with the study. These patients would have to be excluded from the cohort, even though considerable effort may have been exerted to gather data on them up to the point at which they dropped out. Also, it would be necessary to wait until all of the cohort's members had reached each point in time before the probability of surviving to that point could be calculated. Because patients ordinarily become available for a study over a period of time, at any point in calendar time there would be a relatively long follow-up for patients who entered the study first, but only brief experience with those who entered recently. The last patient who entered the study would have to reach each year of follow-up before any information on survival to that year would be available.

Life Table Analysis

In order to make efficient use of all the data, a way of estimating the survival of a cohort over time, called *survival or life table analysis*, is used. Another name for this kind of analysis is the "actuarial method", because it has been used extensively by the insurance industry.

A life table analysis can be depicted graphically, as shown in Figure 7.5. On the vertical axis is the probability of surviving, and on the horizontal axis is the period of time following the beginning of observation. Often the numbers of patients at risk at various points in time are shown, to give some idea of the contribution of chance to the observed rates.

With the life table method, the chance of surviving to any point in time is estimated from the cumulative probability of surviving each of the time intervals that preceded it. Time intervals can be made as small as necessary, even days. For the majority of such intervals, no one dies and the probability of surviving is one. For some, one or more patients die and the probabilities of surviving during those intervals are calculated as the ratio of the number of patients surviving to the number at risk of dying during the interval. Patients who have already died, dropped out, or have not yet been followed-up to that point, are not at risk of dying, and so are not used to estimate survival for the interval. The probability of surviving does not change during intervals in which no one dies; so in practice the probability of surviving is re-calculated only for intervals in which there has been a death. Although the probability assigned to any one of the intervals is not very accurate, because of the small number of events involved, the overall probability of surviving up to each point in time is remarkably accurate.

The life table approach can be used to describe other outcomes of disease besides death—for example, recurrence of tumor, rejection of graft or reinfection. In fact, the frequency of any event can be studied by means of life tables, as long as the event is dichotomous (i.e., either—or), and the event can occur only once during the follow-up period.

Interpreting Survival Curves

Several points must be kept in mind when interpreting survival curves. First, the vertical axis represents the probability of surviving for members of a hypothetical cohort, not the percent surviving for an actual cohort.

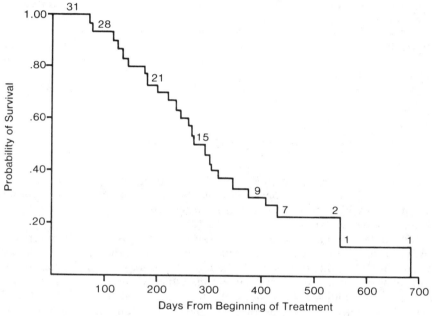

Figure 7.5.   A Survival Curve. The Survival of Patients with Small Cell Carcinoma of the Lung Treated with Combination Chemotherapy. The numbers above the line represent the number of patients at risk at various times. (Data from: Rudnick S. Unpublished.)

In Figure 7.5, 31 patients were observed during the first several weeks. If a cohort of 31 patients was being observed throughout the follow-up period, at a point where 10% had survived (540 days), one would expect 0.10×31 or about 3 patients to be alive. In fact, only one patient is shown to be at risk. The other two were, for one reason or another, not observed for as long as 540 days.

Second, points on a survival curve are the best estimate, for a given set of data, of the probability of survival for members of a cohort. However, confidence in these estimates depends, like all observations on samples, on the number of observations upon which the estimate is based. One can be more confident that the estimates on the *left-hand side* of the curve are sound, because more patients are at risk during this time. But at the tail of the curve, on the *right*, the number of patients upon which estimates of survival are based often becomes relatively small because deaths, drop-outs, and late entrants to the study result in fewer and fewer patients being followed for that length of time. As a result, estimates of survival towards the end of the follow-up period can be strongly affected by what happens to relatively few patients. In Figure 7.5, the probability of surviving is 10% at 680 days. If at that point the one remaining patient happens to die, the probability of surviving would fall to zero. Clearly this would be a too literal reading of the data. Estimates of survival at the tails of survival curves must, therefore, be interpreted with caution.

Finally, the shape of some survival curves, particularly those in which most patients experience the event of interest, gives the impression that patients die rapidly early on, then reach a plateau at which the risk of dying is considerably less. But this impression is deceptive. As time passes, rates of survival are being applied to a diminishing number of people, and this accounts for the smaller slope of the curve.

BIAS IN COHORT STUDIES

Regardless of whether cohort studies are used to study risk or prognosis, bias in their conduct can have the effect of creating apparent differences where none actually exist in nature, or obscuring differences where they really do exist.

The potential for bias exists in cohort studies, just as it does for any observations. Bias can be recognized more easily by those who know where in the course of research it is most likely to occur. They are then in a position to ask important questions which bear on the validity of a study. First, could bias be present under the conditions of the study? Second, is bias actually present in the particular study being considered? Third, are the consequences of bias sufficiently large that they distort the conclusions in a clinically important way? If damage to the study's conclusions is not very great, then the presence of bias may be interesting but is not responsible for misleading results.

Some of the characteristic locations of bias in cohort research are illustrated in Figure 7.6. They should always be considered when evaluating the conclusions of cohort research.

Assembly Bias

Cohort studies are liable to *assembly bias* because when groups of patients are assembled they may differ in ways other than the factors

under study. These unknown or unwanted factors may themselves determine the outcome. If so, observed differences in cohorts at the end of
follow-up may simply reflect differences at the beginning, and not the
particular factors being studied.

Some of the ways in which assembly bias may affect studies of prognosis
include differences among cohorts in the extent of disease, the presence
of other diseases, the time in the course of disease and prior treatment.
The following illustrates how assembly bias was assessed during a study
of patients with Hodgkin's disease.

Example—It has been suggested that patients with Hodgkin's disease have a
worse prognosis if they have a large mediastinal mass when originally diagnosed.

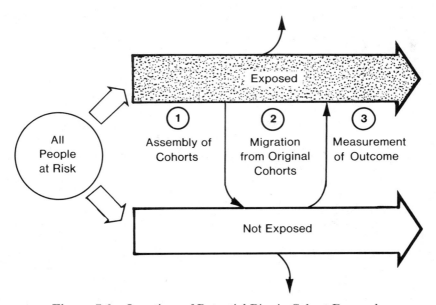

Figure 7.6.   Locations of Potential Bias in Cohort Research.

To investigate this assertion, a study was done of 79 patients with Hodgkin's
disease, all of whom were initially treated with curative-intent nodal irradiation.
Nearly all entered a remission after initial treatment, regardless of the size of the
mass. However, patients who initially had large mediastinal masses had a much
higher relapse rate (74%) than those with small (27%) or no (19%) mediastinal
masses. Could other prognostic factors—particularly initial stage of disease and
symptoms—explain the difference? The authors found that size of mass was
related to relapse rate regardless of the stage of disease, and whether or not there
were symptoms. (Table 7.3) Therefore, size of mediastinal mass was considered
an independent prognostic sign. Assembly bias due to staging and symptoms was
not present (3).

Migration Bias

Migration bias occurs when patients in one cohort move from their original cohort, either to one of the other cohorts under study or out of the study altogether. If these changes take place on a sufficiently large scale, they can affect the validity of conclusions. Migration is another form of selection bias.

In nearly all studies, some members of the original cohort drop out of the study. If these dropouts occur randomly, such that the characteristics of lost subjects in one cohort are on the average similar to those in the other, then no bias would be introduced. This is so whether or not the number of dropouts is similar in the cohorts. But ordinarily the characteristics of lost subjects are not the same in various cohorts. The reasons for dropping out—death, recovery, side effects of treatment, etc.—are often related to prognosis and may also affect one cohort more than

Table 7.3

Analysis of Assembly Bias. The Risk of Recurrence of Hodgkin's Disease According to Size of Mediastinal Mass, Stratified for Stage and Symptoms*

	Size of Mediastinal Mass	
	Large	Small and None
Stage	Recurrence Rate (%)	
II	10/14 (71)	6/32 (19)
III	4/4 (100)	7/13 (54)
Symptoms		
No	10/14 (71)	11/41 (27)
Yes	4/4 (100)	2/4 (50)

* Data from: Lee CK, Bloomfield CD, Goldman AI, Levitt SH. *Cancer*, 1980; 46:2403–2409.

another. As a result, cohorts which were comparable at the outset may become less so as time passes.

Patients may also change over from one cohort to another during their follow-up. Whenever this occurs, the original reasons for subjects falling into one cohort or the other no longer apply. If exchange of patients between cohorts takes place on a large scale, it can diminish the observed difference in risk compared to what might have been observed if the original cohorts had remained intact.

Example—The relationship between exercise and cardiovascular disease was studied by classifying 3975 longshoremen by work activity and observing their rate of fatal heart attacks over a 22-year period. It was recognized that longshoremen originally called active might move to less active jobs, obscuring any relationship that might exist between activity and coronary disease. To deal with this, the investigators re-classified the longshoremen's activity each year, and looked at risk one year at a time. After adjusting for other risk factors, sedentary workers experienced twice the heart attack rate of the most active group (4).

Measurement Bias

Measurement bias is possible if patients in one of the cohorts stand a better chance of having their outcome detected. Obviously some outcomes—like death, cardiovascular catastrophies, or major cancers—are so obtrusive that they are unlikely to be missed. But for less clear-cut outcomes—the specific cause of death, subclinical disease, side effects, or disability—apparent frequency can be biased by differences in the vigor with which they are sought.

Example—In the Framingham Study of coronary heart disease (CHD), "sudden death" was considered due to CHD when it was "documented to have occurred in a matter of minutes and was attributed to no other cause by the physician who completed the death certificate and when no other cause of death was suggested by prior medical history." But there are other causes of dying suddenly, among them subarachnoid hemorrhage, and metabolic and respiratory disturbances. What if it were generally believed, while the study was in progress, that cardiovascular risk factors were related to sudden death? Then physicians completing death certificates, faced with some uncertainty about the actual cause of death, might be more likely to go along with coronary disease as the cause if the deceased had cardiovascular risk factors than if he or she did not. This might artificially inflate the observed relationship between risk factors and sudden death (5).

CONTROLLING FOR BIAS

To determine the effect of a factor on prognosis, ideally we would like to compare cohorts with and without the factor, everything else being equal. But in real life "everything else" is usually not equal in cohort studies.

What can be done about it? There are several possible ways of controlling for differences (Table 7.4). For any observational study, if one or more of these strategies has not been applied, the reader should be skeptical.

Restriction

The patients who are enrolled in a study can be restricted to only those possessing a narrow range of characteristics, so that patients do not vary much, one from the other. For example, the effect of age on prognosis after acute myocardial infarction could be studied in white males with uncomplicated anterior myocardial infarctions. One should keep in mind, however, that while restrictions on entry to a study can certainly produce homogeneous groups, this is at the expense of generalizability. In the course of excluding potential subjects, cohorts may be selected which are unusual, and not representative of most patients with the condition.

Matching

Subjects can be matched as they enter the study so that for each patient in one group there are one or more patients in the comparison group with the same characteristics except for the factor of interest. Often patients are matched for age and sex, because these factors are strongly related to the prognosis of many diseases. But matching for other factors may be called for as well, such as stage or severity of disease, rate of progression, and prior treatments. An example of matching in a cohort study of sickle cell trait was presented under the discussion of observational studies in Chapter 6 (page 96).

Table 7.4
Controlling for Bias when Making Comparisons

Restriction	When selecting participants for a study, limit their range of characteristics
Matching	For each patient in one group, select one or more patients with the same characteristics (except for the one under study) for a comparison group
Stratification	Compare rates within subgroups (strata) of patients with otherwise similar risk
Standardization	Mathematically adjust crude rates so that for the groups being compared equal weight is given to strata of similar risk
Multivariate Adjustment	Adjust for differences in a large number of factors related to outcome, using mathematical techniques
Assuming the Worst	When a factor cannot be controlled, examine the consequences of an unlikely (or worst possible) maldistribution between groups
Randomization	Assign patients to groups in a way that gives each patient an equal chance of falling into one or the other group

Although matching is commonly used, and can be very useful, it controls for bias only for those factors taken into account. Also, it is usually not possible to match for more than a few factors, because of practical difficulties in finding patients who meet all the matching criteria. Moreover, if categories for matching are relatively crude, there may be room for substantial differences between matched groups. For example, if a study of risk for Down's Syndrome were conducted in which there was matching for maternal age within 10 years, there could be a nearly 10-fold difference in frequency related to age if most of the women in one group were 30 and most in the other 39.

Stratification

After data are collected, they can be analyzed and results presented according to sub-groups of patients, or *strata*, of similar characteristics.

Example—Let us suppose we want to compare the operative mortality rates for coronary bypass surgery at Hospitals A and B. Overall, Hospital A noted 48 deaths in 1200 bypass operations (4%) and Hospital B experienced 64 deaths in 2400 operations (2.6%).

The crude rates suggest superiority of B's surgeons. Or do they? Perhaps patients in the two hospitals were not otherwise of comparable prognosis. On the basis of age, myocardial function, extent of occlusive disease, and other characteristics, the patients can be divided into subgroups based on preoperative risk (Table 7.5); then the operative mortality rates within each category or stratum of risk can be compared.

Table 7.5 shows that when patients are divided by preoperative risk, the operative mortality rates in each risk stratum are identical in two hospitals: 6% in high risk patients; 4% in medium risk patients; and 0.067% in low risk patients. The obvious source of the misleading impression created by examining only the crude rates is the important differences in the risk characteristics of the patients

Table 7.5

Example of Stratification. Death Rates after Coronary Bypass Surgery in Two Hospitals, Stratified by Preoperative Risk (Fictitious Data)

Preoperative Risk	Hospital A			Hospital B		
	Patients	Deaths	Rate (%)	Patients	Deaths	Rate (%)
High	500	30	6	400	24	6
Medium	400	16	4	800	32	4
Low	300	2	0.67	1200	8	0.67
Total	1200	48	4	2400	64	2.6

treated at the two hospitals: 42% of A's patients and only 17% of B's patients were high risk.

Stratification is one of the most common and most revealing ways of examining for bias, particularly confounding bias.

Standardization

Two rates can be compared without bias if they are adjusted so as to equalize the weight given to another factor that could influence outcome. This process, called *standardization* (or *adjustment*), shows what the overall rate would be if strata specific rates were applied to a population of similar composition. In the previous example, the high risk mortality rate of 6% receives a weight of 500/1200 in Hospital A and a much lower weight of 400/2400 in Hospital B and so on such that the crude rate for Hospital A equals (500/1200 × 0.06) + (400/1200 × 0.04) + (300/1200 × 0.0067) or 0.04 and the crude rate for Hospital B equals (400/2400 × 0.06) + (800/2400 × 0.04) + (1200/2400 × 0.0067) or 0.026.

If equal weights are used, let us say 1/3 (but they could be anything), then the standardized rate for Hospital A equals $(1/3 \times 0.06) + (1/3 \times 0.04) + (1/3 \times 0.0067)$ or 0.036 which is exactly the same as the standardized rate for Hospital B. The consequence of giving equal weight to strata in each group is to remove totally the apparent excess risk of Hospital A.

The difference between the crude operative mortality rates in the two hospitals results from the bias introduced by the differences in patients' preoperative risk. We are only interested in differences attributable to the hospitals and their surgeons, not to the patients per se. The difference in the crude mortality rates is confounded by the differences in patients while the absence of a difference in the standardized incidence rates is unbiased, unconfounded or controlled.

Multivariate Adjustment

Standardization is the humble forerunner of a modern family of mathematical techniques, generally referred to as multivariate analysis, which have come on the scene in recent years. These techniques give equal weight to a number of variables that could influence outcome. Their advantage is that they can control for baseline differences in a large number of variables at the same time. None of the other strategies can do this. However, these techniques have the disadvantages that they rest on assumptions about the data which are not necessarily true in a given situation. Also, their results are presented in ways that are not readily examined and understood by those of us who are not statisticians.

Assuming the Worst

When data on important factors are not available, it is possible to estimate their effect by assuming the worst possible maldistribution of a factor between the groups being compared and seeing how that would affect rates. For example, to estimate the effect of smoking on coronary heart disease, one would assume that all people in one group smoked, and none in the other, and calculate what the rates would be under these circumstances. In this way, it is possible to see the consequences of the "worst case" effects of smoking.

Assuming the worst is a particularly stringent test of how a factor might affect the conclusions of a study. A less conservative approach is to assume that the factor is distributed between the groups in an unlikely way.

Example—The University Group Diabetes Program (UDGP) study of treatment for mild diabetes found that patients given tolbutamide experienced a greater risk of dying from cardiovascular disease than those given insulin or diet alone. The results were criticized because data on smoking (which is associated with cardiovascular death) were not collected and not taken into account in the analysis. It was suggested that if cigarette smokers were unequally distributed among the groups, such that there were more smokers among those receiving tolbutamide than in the other groups, then the difference in death rates might be related to smoking, not tolbutamide. However, Cornfield has pointed out that even if cigarette smokers in the tolbutamide group exceeded those in the control group by 20%, a situation that would have been extremely unlikely by chance (1/50,000), an increased risk in the tolbutamide group would have persisted. Thus, bias in the distribution of smokers could not have accounted for the observed differences (6).

The "worst case" strategy is used in conjunction with one of the other methods, where either data are missing or in doubt.

All of these ways of dealing with unwanted differences between groups have a limitation. They are effective against only those factors which are known to be related to outcome, and are singled out for consideration. They do not deal with prognostic factors which are not known at the time of the study, or are known but not taken into account.

Randomization

The only way to equalize all factors, known and unknown, is to assign the groups randomly, so that each patient has an equal chance of falling into one or the other group. As we mentioned, it is usually not possible to study prognosis in this way. The special situations in which it is possible to allocate exposure randomly, usually to study the effects of treatment on prognosis, will be discussed in Chapter 8.

The various ways in which meaningful differences between groups being compared, other than the factor of interest, can be controlled are the challenge of cohort studies. A great deal of technology has developed recently to assist in these maneuvers. This should not distract the reader from asking the basic question: are the differences in prognosis in the groups related to the particular factor used to distinguish them or some other factors?

SUMMARY

Prognosis is a description of the course of disease from its onset. Compared to risk, prognostic events are relatively frequent and, often, can be estimated by personal clinical experience. However, cases of disease ordinarily seen in medical centers, and reported in the medical literature, are often biased samples of all cases and tend to overestimate severity.

Prognosis is best described by the probability of having experienced an outcome event at any time in the course of disease. In principle, this can be done by observing a cohort until all who will experience the outcome of interest have done so. However, because this approach is inefficient, another method, called life table analysis, is often used. The onset of events over time is estimated by accumulating the rates for all patients at risk during the preceding time intervals.

As for any observations on cohorts, studies comparing prognosis can be biased if differences arise because of the way cohorts are assembled, whether or not patients remain in their initial cohorts, and whether outcome is assessed equally. A variety of strategies are available to deal with such differences as might arise, so as to allow fair (unbiased) comparisons. One of them should be found whenever comparisons are made.

Suggested Reading

Coldman AJ, Elwood JM. Examining survival data. *Canad Med Assoc J* 1979; 120:1065–1071.

Colton T. Longitudinal studies and use of the life table. *In*: Statistics in Medicine. Chapter 9. Boston: Little, Brown and Co, 1974.

Feinstein AR. Clinical Biostatistics. C. V. Mosby, St. Louis, 1977.

Fries JF, Ehrlich GE. Prognosis. Contemporary Outcomes of Disease. Bowie, Maryland, Prentice Hall, 1981.

Lilienfeld AM. Foundations of Epidemiology. Chapter 9. Prospective Studies. New York: Oxford University Press, 1976.

MacMahon B, Pugh TF. *In*: Epidemiology. Principles and Methods. Chapter 11. Cohort Studies. Boston: Little, Brown and Co., 1970.

Motulsky AG. Biased ascertainment and the natural history of diseases. *N Engl J Med*, 1978; 298:1196–1197.

Murphy EA. Chapter 6. Survivorship functions. *In*: Probability in Medicine. Baltimore; Johns Hopkins University Press, 1979.

Peto R, Pike MC, Armitage P, Breslow NE, Cox DR, Howard SV, Mantel N, McPherson K, Peto J, Smith PG. Design and Analysis of randomized clinical trials requiring prolonged observation of each patient. II. Analysis and examples. *Br J Cancer* 1977; 35:1–39.

References

1. Percy AK, Nobrega FT, Okazaki H, Glattre E, et al. Multiple Sclerosis in Rochester, Minn. A 60-year appraisal. *Arch Neurol*, 1971; 25:105–111.
2. Shapiro S, Goldberg JD, Hutchison GB. Lead time in breast cancer detection and implications for periodicity of screening. *Am J Epid*, 1974; 100:357–366.
3. Lee CK, Bloomfield CD, Goldman AI, Levitt SH. Prognostic significance of mediastinal involvement in Hodgkin's disease treated with curative radiotherapy. *Cancer*, 1980; 46:2403–2409.
4. Brand RJ, Paffenbarger RS, Sholtz RI, Kampert JB. Work activity and fatal heart attack studied by multiple logistic risk analysis. *Am J Epid*, 1979; 110:52–62.
5. Kannel WB, Dawber TR, Kagan A, Revotskie N. Factors of risk in the development of coronary heart disease—six-year follow-up experience. *Ann Intern Med*, 1961; 55:33–50.
6. Cornfield J. The University Group Diabetes Program. A further statistical analysis of the mortality findings. *JAMA*, 1971; 217:1676–1687.

chapter

8

Treatment

Once the nature of a patient's illness has been established and its expected course predicted, the next question is: what can be done about it? Is there a treatment that improves the outcome of disease? This chapter is about ways of deciding whether a well-intentioned treatment does in fact do more good than harm.

IDEAS AND EVIDENCE

Our ideas about what might be useful treatment arise from virtually any activity within medicine.

Some therapeutic hypotheses are suggested by the mechanisms of disease, at the cellular or molecular level. The combination of antibiotics, trimethoprim-sulfamethoxazole, resulted from research on folic acid metabolism. Drugs like cimetidine, corticosteroids, L-dopa, propranolol, and many antimetabolites were discovered through basic biomedical research.

Other hypotheses about the value of treatment have come from astute observations by clinicians. Two recent examples are the discovery that patients with Parkinson's disease, given amantadine to prevent influenza, show improvement in their neurologic status; and reports that colchicine, given for gout, reduces the frequency of attacks of Familial Mediterranean Fever. The value of these treatments was not predicted by an understanding of the mechanism of these diseases, and the ways in which these drugs work are not yet understood.

Ideas about treatment also come from epidemiologic studies of populations. Burkitt observed that colonic diseases are relatively infrequent in African countries, where diet is high in fiber, compared to developed countries where dietary fiber is low. This observation has led to efforts to prevent diseases like irritable bowel syndrome, diverticulitis, appendicitis, and colo-rectal cancer with high fiber diets.

Testing Ideas

Some treatments are so powerful that their value is self-evident, even without formal testing. We do not have reservations about the role of penicillin for pneumonia, surgery for appendicitis, or thyroid hormone replacement for hypothyroidism. Clinical experience has been sufficient.

Usually, however, the effects of treatment are considerably less dramatic. It is then necessary to put ideas about treatments to a formal test, because a variety of conditions—coincidence, faulty comparisons, spontaneous changes in the course of disease, wishful thinking, etc.—can obscure the true relationship between treatment and effect. As Lewis Thomas put it, "Hunches and intuitive impressions are essential for getting the work started, but it is only through the quality of the numbers at the end that the truth can be told" (1).

For some clinical problems our knowledge of disease mechanisms, based on work with cell cultures, experimental animals, and other laboratory models, has become so extensive that it is tempting to predict effects in humans without formal testing. Unfortunately, even for the most well-studied diseases medical knowledge is far from complete. Relying solely on our current understanding of mechanisms, without testing out ideas on intact humans, can lead to unpleasant surprises.

Example—Disseminated herpes zoster is a serious and potentially fatal disease among patients with compromised resistance to infection. The drug cytosine arabinoside (Ara-C) interferes with pyrimidine synthesis, and is inhibitory in vitro against several DNA viruses including the herpes zoster virus. It seemed, therefore, that Ara-C might be useful for treating disseminated zoster. To test this possibility, 39 patients were given either Ara-C or no active drug, and their subsequent course observed. The results are summarized in Table 8.1. Patients receiving Ara-C did worse than those given no specific treatment. One interpretation of these data was that depression of host responses by Ara-C outweighed the drug's antiviral effects, so that no net benefit (and probably some harm) resulted from giving the drug (2).

Therefore, it is almost always necessary to test therapeutic hypotheses by means of clinical research, in which data are collected on the clinical course of patients who have actually experienced the treatment. As one author put it, treatments should be given "not because they ought to work, but because they do work" (3).

TREATMENTS

Treatment is usually considered to be what physicians prescribe—drugs, surgery, etc.,—for patients with established disease. But it should be evident that there are a great many other ways of intervening to improve health (Figure 8.1). One can prevent disease before it is established, by controlling risk factors (*primary prevention*). Disease can be detected early, and treated when it is more likely to respond (*secondary prevention*). Also one can intervene to change the organization of financing health care to render its delivery more effective.

Regardless of the nature of a well-intentioned intervention, the principles by which it is judged superior to its alternatives are the same. Before considering these principles, we will discuss four characteristics of the intervention itself that determine its usefulness to clinicians.

Application in Practice

Is the intervention in question one that is likely to be implemented in usual clinical practice? In an effort to standardize therapy, so as to have

Table 8.1

Formal Testing of a Promising Treatment. The Effect of an Antiviral Agent, Cytosine Arabinoside (ARA-C), on Disseminated Herpes Zoster

	Ara-C (n = 20)	Controls (n = 19)	P
Patients with Virus Dissemination ≥ 6 Days	5	0	0.03
Length of Hospital Stay (Days)	9.4	5.6	0.1
Death	1	0	>.20

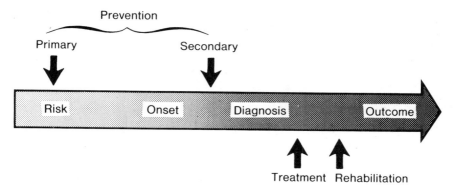

Figure 8.1.   Interventions in the Course of Disease.

it easily described and reproducible in other settings, some investigators end up studying treatments which are so unlike those ordinarily used that the results of the trial are not useful.

Example—Early trials of beta-adrenergic blocking drugs to prevent arrhythmias after acute myocardial infarction used fixed doses of propranolol. But patients vary in their physiologic responses to beta-blockers. It is ordinarily recommended that the dosage of the drug be individualized in order to produce physiologic effects (e.g., slowing of resting pulse and abolition of premature ventricular depolarizations) believed to be good markers of the desired effect (prevention of sudden death). The fixed doses used in the trials were thus contrary to generally accepted recommendations and practice. It is not necessarily wrong to have chosen the fixed doses. But the choice involved a trade-off. In the interest of rigor within the study (internal validity), information was produced that could not be applied readily in practice (4).

Complexity

Single, highly-specific interventions make for good science, because they can be described precisely and applied in a reproducible way. However, clinicians regularly make choices among alternative treatments which involve many elements. Examples include whether to manage a patient with pulmonary edema in an intensive care unit or on the ward; and whether to request chest physiotherapy for patients with respiratory failure or speech rehabilitation for patients with aphasia. All these interventions are amenable to careful evaluation, as long as their essence can be communicated, and reproduced in other settings.

Example—Although most patients with acute myocardial infarction (AMI) are treated in coronary care units (CCUs), evidence that this is the best policy is not conclusive. A study was done, therefore, to determine if there is a difference in early mortality from AMI among patients treated in CCUs, compared to those treated at home.

It was possible to assign 264 patients with suspected AMI to home or hospital care. All patients were visited in their homes, shortly after the onset of symptoms, and a preliminary diagnosis was made. Patients in one group were sent to a regional hospital, where they were admitted to a CCU and cared for in the usual way. The other patients remained at home, and were cared for by their general practitioner.

There was no significant difference in six-week mortality between the home group (13%) and the hospital group (11%). Although the specific components of care in the home and hospital were neither determined by the investigators nor described in detail, it was apparent that these interventions represented care which might ordinarily be given under such circumstances. Thus, the usual policy of admitting all patients to CCUs was not supported, at least for the majority of patients in a community who were suspected of having an AMI (5).

Expected Strength

Is the intervention in question sufficiently different from alternative managements that it is reasonable to expect that outcome will be affected? Some diseases can be reversed by treating a single, dominant cause (e.g., thyroid ablation for hyperthyroidism). But most diseases are determined by a combination of factors acting in concert. Interventions which change only one of them, and only a small amount, cannot be expected to show strong treatment effects. If the conclusion of a trial evaluating such interventions is that a new treatment is not effective, it comes as no surprise.

Example—The Coronary Drug Project was undertaken to determine if decreasing serum lipids by drugs could reduce the risk of coronary heart disease. Men aged 30–64 who had already had one or more myocardial infarctions were randomly allocated to receive a lipid-lowering drug or placebo. In one treatment group, serum cholesterol was about 250 mg % at entry, and fell 16.3 mg % (6.5%) during treatment. After a mean of 74 months of follow-up, there was no difference between treated and control groups in either overall or cause-specific mortality (6).

This trial assessed the effect of a small improvement in one determinant of disease, among patients who already had overt coronary disease. It would have been heartening if a benefit had been found. But the negative results should not be discouraging. The trial did not exclude the possibility that lowering serum lipids substantially, throughout life, would reduce the frequency of coronary disease. The results are even less pertinent to the question: how useful would it be to change several coronary risk factors (e.g., blood pressure, smoking, and cholesterol) together? Such a trial is currently under way.

Obsolescence

Is it possible that changes in patient management have rendered the results of a trial obsolete, even before they become available? Physicians have a tendency to adopt new ways of managing disease, particularly if they make physiologic sense, before they have been rigorously evaluated. Trials take years to complete, and conventional management may have changed substantially while a trial of one component of management is being conducted. Consequently, when the results of a trial become available they are at risk of being considered irrelevant to current medical practice.

We confronted this problem recently during rounds with our housestaff. One of us was discussing a randomized controlled trial, published in 1974, showing that nasogastric suction shortened the course of acute alcoholic pancreatitis (7). After hearing all this, one of our residents objected: 'But we often use cimetidine for pancreatitis and none of these patients was on it. What use is a trial that does not include part of our standard management?" He was right. But cimetidine itself, however attractive a possibility, had not been shown to do more good than harm in acute pancreatitis. At that moment, our management strategies for pancreatitis seemed like the flight plan for a pilot, somewhere over the ocean, who reported to his passengers, "We're lost—but we're making record time!"

CLINICAL TRIALS

Studies of treatment are a special case of studies of prognosis in general, where the particular factor of interest is a therapeutic intervention. Therefore, what has been said about cohort studies (Chapters 6 and 7) applies to studies of treatment as well. Observational studies are in fact one way of assessing treatment. However, because systematic differences in treatment groups occur frequently when they are compared by means of observational studies, it is preferable to impose more order on the comparison.

Clinical trials are a special kind of cohort study in which interventions are specifically introduced by the investigators in ways that improve the possibility of observing treatment effects that are free of bias. The reason for making a distinction between clinical trials and cohort studies is that if the investigator can introduce the intervention, he can also control the conditions of the study in other ways in order to give a more accurate assessment of the effects of an intervention. Clinical trials, thus, are more highly structured than are cohort studies. The investigator is, in effect, conducting an experiment, analogous to those done in the laboratory. He has taken it upon himself (with his subjects' permission) to isolate for study the unique contribution of one factor by holding constant, as much as possible, other determinants of the outcome. Hence, other names for clinical trials are *intervention* or *experimental* studies.

Structure of Clinical Trials

The structure of a clinical trial, in a simplified form, is shown in Figure 8.2. The patients to be studied are first selected from a larger number of patients with the condition of interest. They are then divided into two groups of comparable prognosis. One group, called the *experimental* or treated group, is exposed to some intervention which is believed to be helpful. The other group, called a *control** or comparison group, is treated the same in all ways except that its members are not exposed to the intervention. The clinical course of both groups is then observed, and any differences attributed to the intervention.

The main reason for structuring clinical trials in this way is to avoid bias, or systematic error, when comparing the respective value of the two or more kinds of managements. The validity of clinical trials depends on how well they result in an equal distribution of all determinants of prognosis, other than the one being tested, in treated and control patients.

Of the many factors that can interfere with a fair comparison, five are fundamental (Fig. 8.3).

1. Is a comparison group explicitly identified?
2. Are both treated and control patients selected from the same time and place?
3. Are patients allocated to treated and control groups without bias?
4. Is the intended intervention, and only that intervention, experienced by all of the patients in the treated group, and none in the control group?
5. Is outcome assessed without regard to treatment status?

Depending on the answers to these questions, there are several possible ways of conducting clinical trials.

---

* The term control is used in at least three ways when describing clinical research:

1. In clinical trials, a group which has not received the intervention of interest, and which serves as a standard of comparison when assessing treatment effects.

2. In "case control" studies, a group of patients who do not have the disease in question (Chapter 10).

3. The process of dealing with the effects of extraneous variables (Chapter 7).

UNCONTROLLED TRIALS

Obviously the value of a treatment can only be judged by comparing its results to those of some alternative course of action. The question is

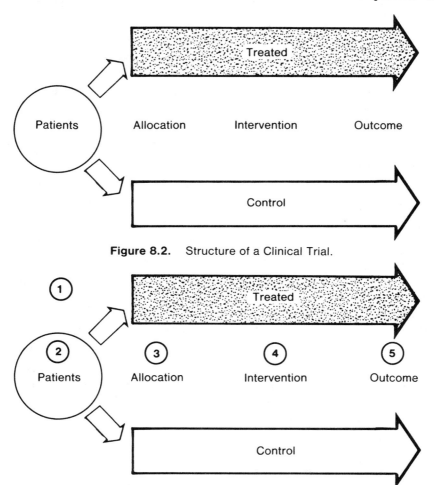

Figure 8.2. Structure of a Clinical Trial.

Figure 8.3. Location of Potential Bias in Clinical Trials. ① Comparison group; ② Patients from same time and place; ③ Unbiased allocation of intervention; ④ Intervention as intended; ⑤ Outcome assessed equally.

not whether a point of comparison is used, but how appropriate it is. In clinical trials, comparison groups can be identified with all degrees of formality—from innuendo to carefully selected, highly comparable controls. Trials are called *uncontrolled* if they specifically describe the course of disease only in a single group of patients who have been exposed to a particular intervention of interest.

What is wrong with assessing the effects of treatment by comparing patients' clinical courses before and after treatment, to see whether an intervention changes the established course of disease in individual patients? The results can be misleading for several reasons.

Unpredictable Outcome

When the clinical course of a disease is quite predictable, a separate control group is less important. We know that subacute bacterial endocarditis left untreated is catastrophic, that most patients with hypothyroidism will only get worse instead of better without exogenous thyroid hormone, and that bowel infarction will not improve without surgery.

However, most therapeutic decisions do not involve diseases with such predictable outcomes. In situations where the clinical course is extremely variable for a given patient, and from one patient to another, assessing treatment effects by using changes in the course of disease after treatment is unreliable.

If the usual course of a disease is to improve, then therapeutic efforts may coincide with improvement but not cause it. For many acute, self-limited diseases—e.g., upper respiratory infections or gastroenteritis—patients tend to seek care when the symptoms are at their worst. They often begin to recover after seeing the doctor because of the natural course of events, and regardless of what was done.

Many severe diseases which are not self-limited, may nevertheless undergo spontaneous remissions in activity which can be misinterpreted as treatment effects. Figure 8.4 shows the clinical course, over a 10-year period, of a patient with systemic lupus erythematosus. Although powerful treatments were not given (because none was available during most of the years shown), the disease passed through dramatic periods of exacerbation, followed by prolonged remissions. Of course, exacerbations like those illustrated are alarming to both patients and doctors, so there is often a feeling that something must be done at these times. If treatment were begun at the peak of activity, improvement would have followed. Without any better comparison than the previous activity of the disease, the treatment would have gotten credit for the improvement.

Hawthorne effect

A great deal of special attention is directed toward patients in clinical trials, and they are well aware of it. Subjects may respond because of the attention, and not because of the treatment itself.

The *Hawthorne effect* is the tendency for people to change their behavior because they are the target of special interest and attention in a study, regardless of the specific nature of the intervention they might be receiving.† It is not clear just what all the reasons for this

---

† The term Hawthorne effect stems from studies done in the 1920's at the Hawthorne Works of the Western Electric Company in Chicago. Workers exposed to varying levels of illumination intensity increased their work output regardless of whether the intensity had

behavior are. But patients are anxious to please their doctors, and make them feel successful. Also, patients who volunteer for trials want to do their part to see that "good" results are obtained.

There is no way of separating out Hawthorne from treatment effects in uncontrolled trials. But if there are control patients who receive the same attention as the treated ones, then the Hawthorne effect cancels out in the comparison.

Regression to the Mean

Treatments are often tried because a manifestation of disease is extreme or unusual—for example, a particularly high blood pressure or fever. In this situation, subsequent measurements may show improvement for purely statistical reasons.

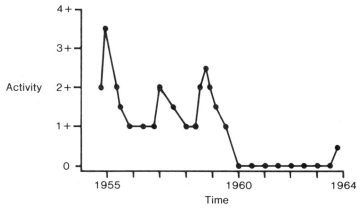

Figure 8.4. The Unpredictable Course of Disease. The Natural History of Systemic Lupus Erythematosus in a Patient Observed Before the Advent of Immunosuppressive Drugs. (Redrawn from: Ropes M. Systemic Lupus Erythematosus. Cambridge: Harvard U. Press, 1976.)

As discussed in Chapter 2, patients selected because they represent an extreme value in a distribution are likely, on the average, to have lower values for later measurements. If those patients are treated after first being found abnormal, and the effects of treatment assessed by subsequent measurements, improvement could be expected even if treatment were ineffective. For the example given in Chapter 2 (p. 38) patients who at first had a mean diastolic blood pressure of 99.2 mm Hg would, even if they were not treated, have had an average fall in blood pressure of 8

increased, decreased or remained the same. It was apparent that characteristics of the study situation other than illumination were responsible for the observed changes. This work is summarized in: Roethlisberger FJ, Dickson WJ, Wright HA. Management and the Worker. Cambridge, MA, 1946.

mm Hg by their next examination. Regression to the mean is therefore another reason why using patients as their own controls can be misleading.

COMPARISONS ACROSS TIME AND PLACE

Time and place are just two ways in which groups of patients being compared can differ. The reason for giving them special consideration is because they are almost always strongly related to prognosis. Clinical trials which attempt to make fair comparisons between groups of patients arising in different eras, or in different settings, have a particularly difficult task.

Time

The results of current treatment are sometimes compared to experience with similar patients in the past—*historical or non-concurrent controls*. While this may be done well, there are many pitfalls. Methods of diagnosis and treatment change with time, and with them the average prognosis.

Example—One approach to assessing the value of coronary care units (CCUs) is to compare death rates of patients hospitalized for acute myocardial infarction in the years prior to CCUs (about 25%) with typical death rates in the current era (about 15%). But more than just CCUs have changed in the interval. More sensitive ways of diagnosing acute myocardial infarctions are also common practice, including lower thresholds for admission of patients with chest pain, and laboratory tests like serum enzymes, nuclear scanning, and continuous ECG monitoring. Because of these changes, the fall in case fatality rates could be attributed to adding mild (good prognosis) cases to the denominator, rather than subtracting deaths from the numerator. This suspicion is supported by recent randomized controlled trials of home versus hospital care, (one of which was cited earlier in this chapter) which do not find an advantage for CCUs for most patients.

If historical controls are used, the shorter the period of time between selection of treated and control groups and the less other aspects of medical care have changed during the interval, the safer an historical control can be. Thus, some oncology centers study a succession of chemotherapeutic regimens by comparing results of the newest regimen to those of the immediately preceding one, often given as recently as the previous year (8). In general, however, choosing *concurrent controls* (i.e., subjects being treated during the same period of time) avoids a potential source of bias.

Place

It is preferable to choose both treated and control patients from the same setting because a variety of factors—referral patterns, organization and skill of staff, etc.—often result in very different prognoses in different settings.

Example—In a study of anticoagulants and acute myocardial infarction, in 22 hospitals the 21-day mortality among patients given anticoagulants, ranged from

0–40% (Figure 8.5). Even if consideration were limited only to those hospitals where there were enough patients included to give a reasonably reliable estimate of death rate, the range was 5.3–21.0%. Differences in mortality rates among hospitals were larger than differences attributed to treatment. If the value of anticoagulants had been studied by comparing death rates in a hospital using anticoagulants, and in another which did not, and the hospitals happened to be ones with quite different death rates in any case, a misleading conclusion would have resulted (9).

ALLOCATING TREATMENT

If it can be accepted that a concurrent control group is preferable, what is the most effective way of assigning patients to receive a new treatment, or serve as controls?

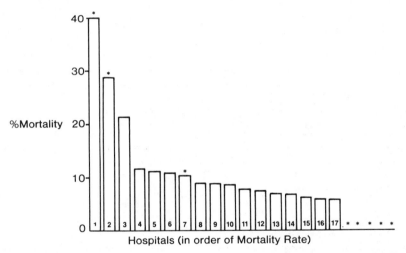

Figure 8.5. Variation in Prognosis by Hospital. The 21-day Mortality From Acute Myocardial Infarction For Patients Treated with Anticoagulants in 22 Hospitals. * Hospitals with <10 Subjects. (Data from: Modan B, Shani M, Schor S, Modan M. *N Engl J Med*, 1975; 292:1359–1362).

Non-random Allocation

One way to allocate patients to treated and control groups is to have the physicians in charge of the patients' care decide. When this is done, the study has all the advantages and disadvantages of cohort studies.

Studies of treated cohorts take advantage of the fact that therapeutic decisions must be made for sick patients regardless of the quality of existing evidence on the subject. In the absence of a clear-cut consensus favoring one mode of treatment over the others, various treatments are often given. As a result, in the course of ordinary patient care, large numbers of patients receive various treatments, and go on to manifest their effects. If experience with these patients can be captured, and properly analyzed, it can be used to guide therapeutic decisions.

Unfortunately, it is often difficult to be sure that observational studies involve unbiased comparisons. Decisions about treatment are determined by a great many factors—severity of illness, concurrent diseases, local preferences, patient cooperation, etc. As a result, patients receiving the various treatments are likely to differ not only in their treatment, but in other ways as well. Efforts to determine the results of treatment alone, free from other factors, are thereby compromised.

Example—There has been a long-standing controversy about whether anticoagulants lower the death rate from acute myocardial infarction (AMI). In one study of this question, the records of 2330 patients treated for AMI in 22 hospitals were reviewed. Physicians had determined which patients received anticoagulants and which did not, using their clinical judgment.

Patients given anticoagulants had a lower 21-day mortality rate than those not receiving such therapy (8.3% versus 27.3%, p < 0.001). The authors noted that the difference in prognosis did not seem related to a variety of prognostic factors including sex, disease severity, site of infarction, diagnostic criteria, or type of hospital.

However, patients not given anticoagulants were older: 65% were at least 60 years old, while only 43% of patients given anticoagulants were this old. Also, patients not given anticoagulants had a much higher mortality rate within the first 48 hours of admission (12.2% versus 1.9%), before anticoagulants could be expected to exert a protective effect, suggesting that they were in general sicker. While these two characteristics, in themselves, do not account for all the difference in mortality, they do establish that there were systematic differences in prognosis in the groups other than whether anticoagulants had been given.

Therefore, it was not possible to reach any firm conclusion in this study about the value of anticoagulants for AMI (9).

Random Allocation

In order to study the unique effects of a clinical intervention, the best way to allocate patients is by means of *randomized controlled trials*, clinical trials in which patients are randomly allocated to treated and control cohorts. Randomization is done by one of a variety of disciplined procedures—analogous to flipping a coin—whereby each subject has an equal chance of appearing in any of the treatment groups.

Random allocation of subjects is preferred because randomization assigns patients to one group or the other(s) without bias. Patients in one group are, on the average, as likely to possess a given characteristic as patients in another. This is so for all factors related to prognosis, whether or not they are known before the study takes place.

However, random allocation is no guarantee that the groups will be similar. While the process of random allocation is unbiased, the results may not be. Dissimilarities between groups can arise, albeit infrequently, by chance alone. The risk of dissimilar groups is particularly great when the number of patients randomized is small. (Consider the likelihood that flipping a coin 10 times will produce heads just half of the time, as opposed to getting very close to 50% heads in the long run, after 1000 tosses.)

To assess whether this kind of "bad luck" has occurred, authors of randomized controlled trials often present a table comparing the frequency of a variety of characteristics in the treated and control groups, especially those known to be related to outcome. It is reassuring to see that important characteristics have, in fact, fallen out nearly equally in the groups being compared. If they have not, it is possible to see what the differences are, and attempt to control them in the analysis (Chapter 7).

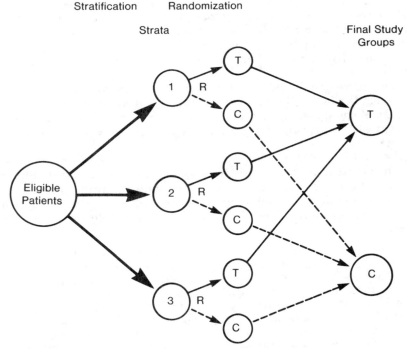

Figure 8.6. Stratified Randomization (*R*) into Treated (*T*) and Control (*C*) Groups.

Stratified Randomization

Some investigators believe it is best to make sure, before randomization, that at least some of the most important characteristics known to be associated with outcome will appear equally in treated and control groups in order to reduce the risk of bad luck. They suggest that patients first be gathered into groups (strata) of similar prognosis and then randomized separately within each stratum (Figure 8.6). The groups are then bound to be comparable, at least for the factors which have been dealt with in this way. Others argue that whatever differences arise by bad luck are unlikely to be large, and can be dealt with mathematically after the data are collected.

REMAINING IN ASSIGNED TREATMENT GROUPS

After patients are allocated to treatment groups, it is intended that they actually take their treatment and remain in their assigned group. But in the real world—even the somewhat rarified real world of clinical trials—a variety of processes tend to disrupt the integrity of the original groups, as constituted just after allocation. Patients may have second thoughts about the treatment they are to receive, and decide the other is really in their best interests. They may also seek other treatment outside the context of the study, fail to follow the prescribed therapeutic regimen, or drop out of the study altogether. Sometimes, patients become seriously ill, causing physicians to change their management or withdraw them from the study.

Under these conditions, cohorts which may have been similar at the outset can become different after randomization has taken place. These differences should either be prevented from arising by diligent efforts on the part of the investigators, or taken into account when the data are analyzed.

When analyzing the results of a trial in which patients have not remained in their original (randomized) groups, a dilemma arises. Should patients who changed treatment groups be counted against the treatment they were originally offered, or the one they ultimately received? The answer depends on the clinical question the trial is intended to answer. As Sackett and Gent have described:

"Trials can ask two different sorts of questions. The first deals with explanations and asks questions such as 'Can Drug A reduce tumor size?' The second deals with management and asks questions such as 'Does prescribing Drug A to patients with tumors do more good than harm?'

These two types of trials have contrasting attributes. The explanatory trial seeks to describe how a treatment produces its effects and to determine whether it can work, often under ideal or restricted circumstances. Conversely, the management trial seeks to describe all the consequences, both good and bad, of treating an illness in a certain way and to determine whether therapy does work, usually under as close to usual clinical circumstances as possible" (10).

Thus, in an explanatory trial, the effects of treatment are analyzed only in those patients who actually receive the treatment, regardless of the group to which they were originally allocated. Conversely, in a management trial, we are interested in the effects of treatment plans, whether they are followed or not, and would compare patient groups according to their original allocation.

It should be evident that when patients are grouped for comparison in any manner other than as originally randomized (for example, as in an explanatory analysis), the advantages of randomization are lost. The groups need no longer be of similar prognosis. This will be discussed later in this chapter.

ASSESSMENT OF OUTCOME

The "cast of characters" for a clinical trial includes three basic actors: those who give treatment (clinicians), those who receive it (patients), and those who assess its effects (investigators). Often the clinicians and investigators are the same people. Participants in a trial may change their behavior in a systematic way (i.e., be biased) if they are aware of which patients receive which treatment.

In general, the more clear-cut the end points used, the less opportunity there is for bias. When the outcome of a trial is measured in unequivocal terms, like being alive or dead, it is unlikely that patients will be misclassified, no matter how biased the assessment of outcome might be. However, for outcomes which are decided by the opinion of one of the participants, there is opportunity for bias. For example, while the fact of death is usually clear, the cause of death is often not. Most persons die for a combination of reasons, or for obscure reasons, allowing some room for judgment in assigning cause of death. This judgment can be influenced by knowledge of what went before, including the treatments that were given. Opportunities for bias are even greater when assessing symptoms like pain, nausea, or depression.

To avoid bias, participants in a clinical trial can be "blinded" in a figurative sense, to knowledge of treatment. That is, efforts can be made to keep them unaware of the treatments individual patients have received.

Blinding Patients

Most patients are anxious to please their physicians, and to get well. This leads to difficulty when assessment of outcome is heavily dependent on what patients report. They may exaggerate their improvement if they know they have received a specific treatment.

To avoid bias from this source, an effort is made to conceal from patients the treatment they are actually receiving. Control patients are given a *placebo:* an intervention which is indistinguishable from the "active" treatment, but does not possess its specifically active component. For example, a placebo pill would be the same size, shape, color, and taste as the active drug. In one study of a surgical procedure for angina pectoris, investigators even went so far as to do a sham operation, including anesthesia and a skin incision! When placebos are successful, it becomes impossible for patients' responses to be biased by knowledge of their treatments.

The process of blinding patients can be more difficult in practice than it might seem in theory. Many medications cause characteristic side effects—e.g., flushing and headache with nitrites, euphoria with opiates, smell with paraldehyde, stain with coal tar—that cannot be disguised.

Blinding Investigators

If the outcomes of alternative treatments are not assessed with equal vigor, and by equal standards, the resulting comparison can be biased. Fortunately, most clinical investigators are honest. But they do believe strongly in their work. Moreover, they are more likely to be rewarded for demonstrating successful than unsuccessful treatments in that it is easier to publish studies with positive results. It may be difficult, therefore, for investigators to avoid unintended bias. They may also want to find ways of protecting themselves from accusations of bias, even when they are confident that none exists.

The most effective way for investigators to avoid bias when assessing outcome is by assuring that they cannot know which treatment any individual patient has received. Among the ways in which investigators can be blinded is by exposing control patients to a placebo, in the manner described in the previous section.

Just as it may be difficult to blind patients, so it may be difficult to blind investigators. In a trial of surgical versus medical management of angina pectoris, even a rather dull physician might suspect that a patient with a large scar over his sternum had received surgery. Similarly, radiotherapy leaves tell-tale skin changes, and chemotherapy may cause alopecia. In situations where assessment cannot be done with blinding, it is incumbent on the investigators to set out firm ground rules describing just how outcomes will be decided and then to follow these rules to the letter.

Placebo Effects

Most medical interventions have both specific and non-specific effects. Because of this, patients given placebos may experience improvement which is over and above what they would have experienced if they had been given nothing at all.

The *placebo effect* is a response to a medical intervention which is definitely a result of the intervention, but not because of its specific mechanism of action.

Example—Patients with chronic severe itching were entered in a trial of antipruritic drugs. During each of three weeks, 46 patients received in random order either cyproheptadine HCl (Periactin), trimeprazine tartrate (Temaril), or placebo. There was a one-week rest period, randomly introduced into the sequence, in which no pills were given. Results were assessed without knowledge of medication, and expressed as "itching scores" (Table 8.2). The two active drugs and placebo were all similarly effective. Both drugs and placebo gave much better results than when nothing at all was given (11).

Placebo-controlled trials are intended to establish whether treatment is valuable over and above what might be achieved by a simpler (placebo) treatment, and not whether treatment is valuable at all. It is important to distinguish the specific from non-specific effects of a treatment in order to know whether the additional cost, risk, and effort of a specific treatment is worthwhile.

Table 8.2
The Placebo Effect. Control of Chronic Itching by Two "Active Drugs" and a Placebo, Compared to No Treatment (36 Patients)*

Drug	Itching Score†
Cyproheptadine HCl	27.6
Trimeprazine Tartrate	34.6
Placebo	30.4
Nothing	49.6

* Data from: Fisher RW. *JAMA*, 1968; 203:418–419.
† The higher the score, the more the itching.

SUBGROUPS

The principal result of a clinical trial is a description of the most important outcome in each of the major treatment groups. But it is tempting to examine the results in more detail than the overall conclusions afford. We begin to look at subgroups of patients with special characteristics, or for particular outcomes. In doing so, however, there are some risks which are not a feature of examining the principal conclusions alone.

Inadequate Number of Patients

Trials which are large enough to answer the principal questions may be far too small to answer more detailed ones.

Example—In the VA Trial of the treatment of hypertension (diastolic blood pressure 115–129 mm Hg), there was a statistically significant reduction in morbid events in the treated group. In all, 27 severe complicating events developed among patients given placebo, and only two among patients given antihypertensive drugs (p < .001).

The general conclusions were accepted, but more specific questions were raised. Did treatment prevent myocardial infarctions? What about renal failure, or retinopathy? These questions could not be answered with confidence because there were simply not enough patients in the study. A total of 143 treated and control patients was sufficient to answer the overall question of benefit. But when the rates of specific events were examined, comparisons involved very small numbers (Table 8.3). For example, only two untreated patients had worsening renal function, and none in the treated group; three untreated patients had dissecting aneurysms, and none of the treated; and so on.

Clearly each of these individual findings could have easily arisen by chance, although the overall distribution of complication—27 versus 2—was very unlikely to be by chance alone (12).

Because examining subgroups in a clinical trial—either certain kinds of patients or specific kinds of outcomes—involves a great reduction in the data available, it is frequently impossible to come to firm conclusions.

Nevertheless, the temptation to look is there, and some tentative information can be gleaned.

Bias

Subgroups of patients that are selected because of characteristics that arise after treatment has been allocated may not be comparable, even if they are taken from groups which were initially unbiased (e.g., ones which had been randomly allocated).

Example—During a large study of the effects of several lipid-lowering drugs on coronary heart disease, 1103 men were given clofibrate and 2789 men were given placebo. The five-year mortality rate was 20.0% for the clofibrate group and 20.9% for the placebo group, indicating that the drug was not effective.

It was recognized that not all patients took their medications. Was clofibrate

Table 8.3

The Paucity of Data in Subgroups. The Occurrence of Severe, Complicating Events in Men With Diastolic Blood Pressure Averaging 115–129 mm Hg, Treated with Antihypertensive Drugs or Placebo*

Event	Number	
	Placebo (N = 70)	Treated (N = 73)
Retinopathy	9	
Heart Disease	4	
Cerebrovascular Disease	4	1
Increasing Hypertension	3	
Aortic Dissection or Aneurysm	3	
Azotemia	3	
Sudden Death	1	
Depression		1
Total	27	2

* Data from: Veterans Administration Cooperative Study Group on Antihypertensive Agents. *JAMA*, 1967; 202:1028–1034.

effective among patients who actually took the drug? The answer appeared to be yes. Among patients receiving clofibrate, five-year mortality for patients taking most of their prescribed drug was 15.0%, compared to 24.6% for the less cooperative patients ($p < 10^{-5}$). However, taking the prescribed drug was also related to lower mortality rates among patients prescribed placebo. For them, five-year mortality was 15.1% for patients taking most of their placebo medication, and 28.3 for patients who did not ($p < 10^{-15}$). It was apparent that there was an association between drug taking and prognosis which was not related to clofibrate.

The authors cautioned against evaluating treatment effects in subgroups determined by patient responses to the treatment protocol after randomization (13).

When experience with subgroups of patients in a clinical trial is presented, it should be treated like the results of any other non-randomized study. It is necessary to look for systematic differences in the groups being compared, and correct for them if they are found.

Chance Associations

When a large number of subgroups are examined, there is an increased chance that one of them will seem to show a statistically significant difference, even if no differences really exist. This problem will be discussed in Chapter 9.

PUBLICATION

Like everyone else, physicians prefer good news. Thus, words like "efficacy," "predicting," "detecting," and "correlation" are the order of the day in journal titles. It is, on the other hand, considerably less appealing to contemplate things that do not work. In fact, such observations are often considered failures. Researchers with the bad fortune to make such observations are likely to be advised by their friends, with gentle malice, to seek publication in the "Journal of Negative Results."

It may be that our penchant for positive results leads to bias in the kinds of articles selected for publication in medical journals. Consider a population of all potential articles, the results of all research carried to completion. Of these, some will find no effect. These negative studies might be less likely to be submitted for publication, because their results are often regarded as less interesting. Of the articles submitted for publication, a larger proportion of those with negative results might be rejected by the editorial process, for the same reason. The outcome of this sequence would be that articles actually reaching publication are a biased sample of all research findings, tending to represent treatments as being more effective than they actually are.

We know of no empiric evidence for publication bias. Certainly there is no reason to assert that biased judgments are made deliberately. Everyone does his part to put the "best" work forward. But publication is not a random process. There are forces favoring positive over negative results which are quite independent of their relative proportions among all research projects undertaken. Readers should be aware of this bias, lest they become unrealistically impressed with the many new and promising findings that appear in medical journals.

One way to avoid this bias is to give more credibility to large studies than to small, because most large studies, having required great effort and expense in their execution, will be published regardless of whether they have a positive or negative finding. Smaller studies, requiring less investment, are more easily discarded in the selection process.

EFFICACY AND EFFECTIVENESS

Patients in clinical trials are often highly selected to cooperate with the medical regimen being evaluated. But ordinary patients are not, and if they fail to follow medical advice they may experience lower success rates for treatment than are reported in clinical trials. A trial's results, thus, are judged in reference to two broad questions: can the treatment work under ideal circumstances? Does it work in ordinary settings? The words efficacy and effectiveness have been applied to these concepts.‡

Efficacy

The question of whether a treatment can work is one of efficacy. An *efficacious* treatment is one that does more good than harm among those who receive it. Efficacy is established by restricting patients in a study to those who will cooperate fully with medical advice.

Example—Figure 8.7 shows how patients were selected for the Veterans' Administration trial of antihypertensive treatment (12). Every effort was made to include only those patients who were fully cooperative, and likely to remain so. As a result, the study itself was tightly constructed and its conclusions well supported. But do the conclusions apply to hypertensive patients in general? Probably not. The authors chose to answer whether antihypertensive medications were helpful under the best possible circumstances. In so doing, they sacrificed generalizability of the results to patients in more ordinary circumstances.

Effectiveness

An *effective* treatment does more good than harm in those to whom it is offered. Effectiveness is established by offering a treatment or program to patients and allowing them to accept or reject it as they might ordinarily do. Only a small proportion of clinical trials set out to answer questions of effectiveness. If a treatment is found to be ineffective, it may be due to lack of efficacy, lack of patient acceptance, or both.

Compliance

Compliance is the extent to which patients follow medical advice. Some have preferred the term "adherence", because it has a less dictatorial connotation. Compliance intervenes between an efficacious treatment and an effective one.

Although non-compliance suggests a kind of willful neglect of good advice, other factors also contribute. Patients may misunderstand which drugs and doses are intended, run out of prescription medications, confuse various (generic) preparations of the same drug, or have no money or insurance to pay for drugs. Taken together, these may limit the usefulness of treatments which have been shown to be efficacious under specially favorable conditions.

Compliance is particularly important in medical care outside the hospital. In the hospital, many factors act to constrain patients' personal behavior and render them compliant. Hospitalized patients are generally

---

‡ The distinction between efficacy and effectiveness is not found in the dictionary. These words have been given specific meanings in order to express important concepts in medical care.

sicker and more frightened. They are in strange surroundings, dependent on the skill and attention of the staff for everything—even their life. What is more, doctors, nurses, and pharmacists have developed a well-organized system for assuring that patients receive what is ordered for

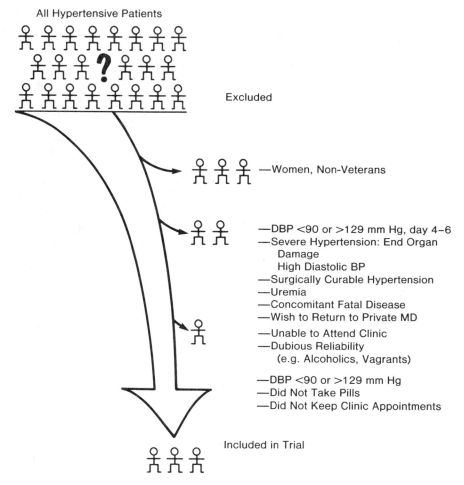

Figure 8.7. Sampling of Patients for a Clinical Trial. The Veterans' Administration Trial of Antihypertensive Therapy. (From Veterans Administration Cooperative Study Group on Antihypertensive Agents *JAMA* 1967; 202:1028–1034).

them. As a result, clinical experience and a medical literature developed on the wards may underestimate the importance of compliance outside the hospital, where most patients and doctors are, and where patients have much greater freedom of choice.

ETHICS

Patients and physicians who become involved in clinical trials often find they are not entirely comfortable with the experience. The various trappings of sound clinical trials—control groups, random allocation of treatment, and blindness—seem like very severe constraints compared to the options available in most doctor-patient encounters, where the sole objective is patient care.

Withholding The "Best" Treatment

Some critics of clinical trials are concerned that patients may not be offered the best possible treatment, according to current knowledge. In fact, trials are not considered ethical if there is already good evidence that one of the treatments is superior. But if it is really not known which is better, how can it be wrong to give one treatment rather than the other? It might even be argued that it is wrong to give a treatment which is not known to be efficacious.

Acceptance Before Evidence

Not infrequently, treatments become firmly ensconced in our therapeutic armamentarium before they have been subjected to sound evaluation by means of controlled clinical trials. This problem is less likely to occur for new drugs, because the Food and Drug Administration requires evidence of safety and efficacy before licensing pharmaceuticals. On the other hand, new technology and surgical procedures are not subject to much regulation, and often come into general use before controlled clinical trials have been undertaken. In fact, new procedures can become so much a part of usual practice that it is virtually impossible to conduct a trial of them. Examples of treatments which have become conventional in the absence of controlled trials include coronary care units, radical mastectomy, and Caesarian section for fetal distress.

Because of this problem, some physicians have advocated "randomization from the first patient" after a new treatment is introduced. Others argue that it is better to conduct rigorous clinical trials somewhat later, after the best way to deliver the treatment has been worked out, so that a good example of the intervention is tested. In any case, it is generally agreed that if a controlled trial is postponed too long, the opportunity to do it at all may be lost.

Informed Consent

Over the past few decades, a growing number of safeguards have been developed so that patients are not used for experiments against their will. Physicians have considerable power over sick people, particularly when patients are in an unusually dependent position—for example, when they are desperately ill, prisoners, or relatively unsophisticated. Also, some physicians have abused their power in the name of gaining new knowledge. How, then, can we ask patients to participate in clinical trials in a way that they can refuse and, if they accept, in a way that protects their rights?

At the present time, proposals for research involving humans must pass a "Committee for the Protection of Human Subjects." Members represent various disciplines within the sponsoring institution, and are not directly involved in the proposed research. Particular attention is given to assuring that patients are not exposed to undue risk (relative to

Table 8.4

Elements of Consent Forms for Human Subjects in Research.*

1. The consent form should not be a "standard form" but must relate to the particular research activity.
2. The consent form must be in language that the subject can understand.
3. Consent forms should be consistent with the legal requirements of the State.
4. The following statement must be included (by Federal and local regulations): "I understand that in the event of physical injury directly resulting from the research procedures, financial compensation cannot be provided. However, every effort will be made to make available to me the facilities and professional skills of the Medical Center."
5. A statement that the study includes research.
6. An explanation of the procedures to be followed.
7. A description of the benefits (if any) to be reasonably expected.
8. A description of the discomforts and risks to be reasonably expected.
9. A disclosure of any alternative procedures which might be advantageous to the subject.
10. A statement describing confidentiality.
11. Instruction to the subject that he/she is free to withdraw without penalty from the research activity at any time.
12. A statement of any additional costs to the subjects.
13. The name of the principal investigator or his/her delegate who is directly responsible for the subject.
14. Instruction to the subject that he/she may contact the present Chairman of the Committee on the Protection of the Rights of Human Subjects, (name and telephone number) if the subject feels that there is any infringement upon his/her rights.
15. If reviewed or sponsored by the FDA, a statement should be included that the FDA may review all records.
16. Consent of a suitable representative if the subject cannot legally represent himself/herself.
17. Signature of witness and date.

* Adapted from the form in use at the University of North Carolina.

the usual care for their condition), and that they have given informed consent for their participation. Table 8.4 shows the elements of informed consent used at our institution. The document meets Federal regulations for human research, and similar requirements are used in institutions throughout the United States.

Unfortunately, there is reason to question whether signing a consent form really means a subject has understood its stipulations. Legal documents notwithstanding, informed consent still rests largely on the ability of investigators to communicate honestly and fully with their subjects.

Clinical trials are undoubtedly awkward to conduct. But as a society, we have little choice. If some patients do not participate in trials, then all patients will be treated without the best possible evidence that more good than harm is being accomplished.

THE REAL WORLD

Randomized controlled trials are the best available means of assessing the value of treatment. However, there are many situations in which

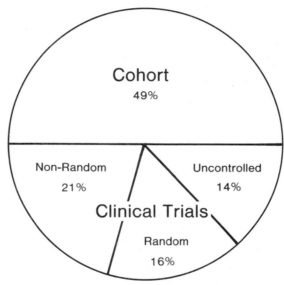

Figure 8.8. Research Design for Articles about Treatment, Published 1966–1976. For: *N Engl J Med, Lancet,* and *JAMA.* (Fletcher SW, Fletcher RH, Greganti MA. *In:* Roberts EB, Levy RI, Finkelstein SN, Moskowitz J, Sondik EJ (Ed). Biomedical Innovations. Cambridge MA: MIT Press, 1981.

treatment cannot be assessed by randomized controlled trials, because of the practical disadvantages of this method. Patients or physicians may refuse to leave to chance which treatment they will use, because they are uncomfortable selecting treatment for individuals with such detachment, or because they may already believe that one treatment is better than the other. Clinical trials are expensive, not infrequently costing millions of dollars per trial. They take time, and our society is not inclined to suspend judgment on promising treatments for long. They require a relatively large number of subjects and in order to assemble them, it is often necessary to conduct a study at several institutions. They are subject to ethical controversies which show no signs of resolution as time passes. Finally, they tend to be rigid, selecting unusual patients and exposing them to modes of care which are not easily duplicated in practice.

Because of many practical difficulties with randomized controlled clinical trials, the majority of therapeutic questions are answered by other means, particularly uncontrolled and non-randomized trials (Figure 8.8).

Partly for a lack of substantial evidence there remains a great deal of controversy about the value of many everyday clinical treatments. There has been vigorous, sometimes acrimonious debate over the effects of "tight" blood sugar control on the chronic complications of diabetes; the ability of bypass surgery to prolong life in patients with coronary disease; and the best surgical procedure for breast cancer—to name just a few.

Although randomized controlled trials are certainly expensive and difficult, their alternative—patient care without sound guidelines—may be more so. Each year, billions of dollars are spent on diagnostic and therapeutic efforts which are of uncertain value. Under the circumstances, properly designed and timely clinical trials could save money.

SUMMARY

Preventive and therapeutic interventions include actions that are intended to change the clinical course of disease for the better. Although many seem like they ought to work, fewer actually do when put to a formal test.

In general, evaluation of treatment is less likely to be biased if the investigator can establish the conditions of treatment in a clinical trial. A comparison (control) group of patients should be explicitly identified, because the clinical course of disease is often not predictable. If treated and control patients are taken from the same time and place, it is possible to avoid a variety of factors other than treatment that can affect outcome. Patients should be allocated into treated and control groups in such a way that they would have the same outcomes if it were not for the treatment. The surest way to do this is randomization. It is preferable (though not always possible) to arrange that participants in a trial are blind (i.e., unaware of individual patients' treatment) so that knowledge of treatment cannot effect their responses. In sum, the soundest approach to a clinical trial is a randomized, double-blind, controlled trial.

The extent to which the results of a clinical trial can be applied to other patients depends on how patients were sampled for inclusion in the trial. On the one hand, efficacy is established in highly cooperative patients, and shows whether an intervention can work under specially favorable circumstances, although not necessarily in practice. On the other hand, effectiveness is whether treatment (prevention) does more good than harm in those to whom it is offered.

Suggested Readings

Wulff HR. *In:* Rational Diagnosis and Treatment. Chapters 9 and 10. Our Therapeutic Legacy; The Controlled Therapeutic Trial. Oxford: Blackwell Scientific Publications, 1976.

Feinstein AR. Section one: The Architecture of Cohort Research. *In* Clinical Biostatistics. St. Louis: C.V. Mosby, 1977.

Peto R, Pike MC, Armitage P, Breslow NE, Cox DR, Howard SV, Mantel N, McPherson K, Peto J, Smith PG. Design and analysis of randomized clinical trials requiring prolonged observations of each patient. *Br J Cancer*, 1977; 34:585–612, 35:1–39.

Byar DP, Simon RM, Friedewald WT, Schlesselman JJ, DeMets DL, Ellenberg JH, Gail MH, Ware JH. Randomized clinical trials. *N Engl J Med*, 1976; 295:74–80.

Gehan EA, Freireich EJ. Non-randomized controls in cancer clinical trials. *N Engl J Med*, 1974; 290:198–203.

Hills M, Armitage P. The two-period cross-over trial. *Br J Clin Pharm*, 1979; 8:7–20.

Sackett DL, Gent M. Controversy in counting and attributing events in clinical trials. *N Engl J Med*, 1979; 301:1410–1412.

Ritter JM. Placebo controlled, double-blind clinical trials can impede medical progress. *Lancet*, 1980; 1:1126–1127.

Relman AS. The ethics of randomized clinical trials: two perspectives. *N Engl J Med*, 1979; 300:1272.

Hill AB. Medical ethics and controlled trials. *Br Med J*, 1963; 1:1043–1049.

References

1. Thomas L. Biostatistics in medicine. *Science*, 1977; 198:675.
2. Stevens DA, Jordan GW, Waddell TF, Merigan TC. Adverse effect of cytosine arabinoside on disseminated zoster in a controlled trial. *N Engl J Med*, 1973; 289:873–878.
3. Opie on the heart. *Lancet*, 1980; 1:692.
4. Ritter JM. Placebo-controlled, double-blind clinical trials can impede medical progress. *Lancet*, 1980; 1:1126–1127.
5. Hill JD, Hampton JR, Mitchell JRA. A randomized trial of home versus hospital management for patients with suspected acute myocardial infarction. *Lancet*, 1978; 1:837–841.
6. Coronary Drug Project Research Group. Clofibrate and niacin in coronary heart disease. *JAMA*, 1975; 231:360–381.
7. Levant JA, Secrist DM, Resin H, Sturdevant RAL, Guth PH. Nasogastric suction in the treatment of alcoholic pancreatitis. A controlled study. *JAMA*, 1974; 229:51–52.
8. Gehan EA, Freireich EJ. Non-randomized controls in cancer clinical trials. *N Engl J Med*, 1974; 290:198–203.
9. Modan B, Shani M, Schor S, Modan M. Reduction of hospital mortality from acute myocardial infarction by anticoagulant therapy. *N Engl J Med*, 1975; 292:1359–1362.
10. Sackett DL, Gent M. Controversy in counting and attributing events in clinical trials. *N Engl J Med*, 1979; 301:1410–1412.
11. Fischer RW. Comparison of antipruritic agents administered orally. *JAMA*, 1968; 203:418–419.
12. Veterans Administration Cooperative Study Group on Antihypertensive Agents. Effects of treatment on morbidity in hypertension. II. Results in patients with diastolic blood pressure averaging 90 through 114 mm Hg. *JAMA*, 1967; 202:1028–1034.
13. The Coronary Drug Project Research Group. Influence of adherence to treatment and response of cholesterol on mortality in the coronary drug project. *N Engl J Med*, 1980; 303:1038–1041.

chapter

9

Chance

selection
measure
confounding

When physicians attempt to learn from clinical experience, whether observed during formal research or in the course of patient care, their efforts are impeded by two processes: bias and chance.

As we have discussed, bias is systematic error—anything which results in observations which systematically differ from the true values. When clinical research is done, a great deal of the effort is aimed at avoiding bias where possible, and dealing with bias when it is unavoidable. It is at least theoretically possible to design research which avoids bias altogether—for example, by a perfect double-blind, randomized, placebo-controlled trial.

Chance, on the other hand, is inherent in all observations. It can be minimized but never avoided altogether. Chance is the result of random variation arising from either the process of measurement itself or the biologic phenomenon being measured. This source of error is called "random" because on the average it is as likely to result in observed values being on one side of the true value as on the other.

Most of us tend to be impressed by statistics, and thereby risk overestimating the importance of chance, compared to bias, when interpreting data. We might say, in essence, "If p is <0.001, a little bit of bias can't do any harm!" But if data are assembled with unrecognized bias, no amount of statistical elegance can save the day.

In this chapter, chance will be discussed in the context of a controlled clinical trial, because that is a simple way of presenting the concepts. However, it should be noted that application of the concepts developed is not limited to comparisons of treatments in clinical trials. Statistics apply whenever one makes inferences about populations based on information obtained from samples.

STATISTICAL TESTS

When a clinical trial is done, the observed differences between treated and control subjects cannot be expected to represent the true differences exactly, because of random variation in both of the groups being compared. Statistical tests help to make inferences about the true state of affairs. Why not measure the true state of affairs directly and do away with this uncertainty? The reason is that research must ordinarily be conducted on a sample of patients, and not all patients with the condition under study. As a result, there is always a possibility that the particular sample of patients in a study, even though selected in an unbiased way, might not be representative of the whole. One professional statistician explained it this way:

A statistical test is simply a tool to help an investigator bridge the gap between observed sample results and hypothesized universe states. An investigator wishes to draw conclusions about a particular group of objects. In medical research, these are usually patients with a particular characteristic. In many research projects, the entire group about which conclusions are to be drawn is not available for the experiment. The investigator must then perform his experiment on a "sample" from his "target population." He can make decisions about the target population after looking at his sample results by guessing, by relying on his experience, or by calculating appropriate probabilities in terms of the manner in which the experiment was carried out. The probabilities so calculated are what many people refer to as "statistical tests" (1).

In the usual situation, where the principal conclusions of a trial are expressed in dichotomous terms, (i.e., the treatment was either successful or not) there are four ways in which those conclusions might relate to reality (Figure 9.1).

Two of the four possibilities lead to correct conclusions. These are when the treatments really do have different effects, and that is the conclusion of the study; and when the treatments really have the same effects, and the study concludes this is so.

There are also two ways of being wrong. The treatments under study may be actually no better than no treatment, but it is concluded that the study treatment is better. Error of this kind, resulting in a "false positive" conclusion that the treatment is effective, is referred to as α or *Type I* error. Alpha is the error of saying there is a difference when there is not. On the other hand, treatment might be effective but the study concludes that it is not. This "false negative" conclusion is called a β or *Type II* error. Beta is the error of saying there is no difference when there is.

The reader may recognize that Figure 9.1 is similar to the four-fold table comparing the results of a diagnostic test to the true diagnosis (Chapter 3). Here the "test" is the conclusion of a clinical trial, based on a statistical test of results from a sample of patients. Reality is the true relative merits of the treatments being compared, if they could be established for all patients with the illness under study. The α error is analogous to a false positive and β error to false negative test result. In the absence of bias, random variation is responsible for the uncertainty of the statistical conclusion.

Because random variation plays a part in all observations, it is an oversimplification to ask whether or not chance accounted for the results. Rather, it is a question of how likely random variation is to have determined the findings under the particular conditions of the study. The probability of error due to random variation is estimated by means of *inferential statistics*, a quantitative science which, based on assumptions

	True Difference	
	Present	Absent
Conclusion of Statistical Test — Different	Correct	Incorrect (Type I or α error)
Conclusion of Statistical Test — Not Different	Incorrect (Type II or β error)	Correct

Figure 9.1. The Relationship Between the Results of a Statistical Test and the True Difference between Two Treatments.

about the mathematical properties of the data, allows calculations of the probability that the results could have occurred by chance alone.

Statistics are more than a little awesome to most of us. The field has its own jargon—e.g., variance, regression, universe, power—that is considered exotic by most clinicians. Also, statistics rely on math—or worse, computers—to get the answers! Confronted with all this, apparently so foreign to medicine, it is easy for a clinician to be intimidated. However, leaving aside the genuine complexity of statistical method, inferential statistics should be regarded by the non-expert as a useful means to an end. Statistics are the means by which the effects of random variation are estimated.

The succeeding two sections will discuss α and β error, respectively. We will attempt to place inferential statistics, as they are used to estimate the probabilities of these errors, in context. No attempt will be made to deal with these subjects in a rigorous, quantitative fashion. For that, the reader is referred to a number of excellent textbooks of biostatistics (see Suggested Readings.)

CONCLUDING A TREATMENT WORKS

Most of the inferential statistics encountered in the current medical literature express the likelihood of an α error by means of the familiar p value. The p value is a quantitative statement of the probability that observed differences in the particular study at hand could have happened by chance alone, assuming that there is in fact no difference between the groups in the long run. Another way of expressing this is that p is an answer to the question; if there were no difference between treatments and the trial were repeated many times, what proportion of the trials would lead to the conclusion that a treatment is effective?

We will call the p value "p_α" to distinguish it from estimates of the other kind of error due to random variation, β error, which we will refer to as p_β. It should be evident that the kind of error estimated by p_α applies when the conclusion is drawn that one treatment is more effective than another. If it is concluded that there is no difference between treatments, then p_α is not relevant. In that situation, p_β (probability of β error) applies.

It has become customary to attach special significance to p values falling below 0.05. This is because it is generally agreed that one chance in twenty is a small risk of being wrong. One in twenty is so small, in fact, that it is reasonable to conclude such an occurrence is unlikely to have arisen by chance alone. It could have arisen by chance, and one in twenty times it will. But it is unlikely.

Differences associated with p_α less than 0.05 are often called "statistically significant." It is important to remember, however, that setting a cut-off point at 0.05 is entirely arbitrary. Reasonable people might accept higher values, or insist on lower ones, depending on the consequences of a false positive conclusion in a given situation.

To accommodate various opinions about what is and is not unlikely, some experts prefer that the actual probabilities of an α error be reported—e.g., 0.03, 0.07, 0.11, etc.—rather than lumping them into two categories, <0.05 or ≥0.05. The interpretation of what is statistically significant is then left to the reader. However, p values greater than one in five are usually reported as simply p_α >0.20 because nearly everyone can agree that a risk of random error which is greater than one in five is an unacceptably high risk.

Some statisticians prefer that the contribution of chance to observed differences be expressed as *confidence intervals*. A confidence interval is a range of values selected in such a way that there is a specified probability (usually 0.95 or 19/20) of including the true value. Reporting means, with confidence intervals, puts the emphasis where it belongs: on the magnitude of observed differences. The observed difference is, after all, our best estimate of the true difference. Adding confidence intervals conveys a picture of how far from the true value the observed difference could lie because of random variation.

Example—Figure 9.2 illustrates confidence intervals for a study of the risk of carcinoma of the pancreas related to coffee drinking. Assuming no bias, the data show a relative risk of 2.3 for women and 2.6 for men, and these are the best estimates of the true relative risks. However, the confidence intervals are broad the results are consistent with a risk as large as 5.4 and as small as 1.2, almost no risk at all. Of course, if there was bias in the conduct of this study, the observed risks could be even further from the true ones (2).

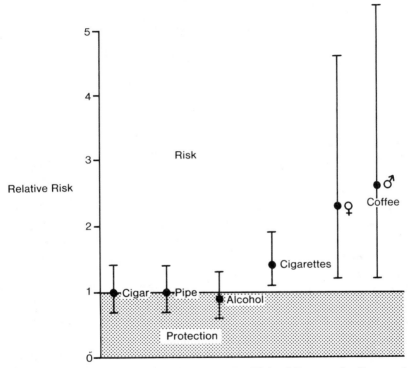

Figure 9.2.   Example of Confidence Intervals. Risk of Pancreatic Cancer Associated with Exposure to Several Factors. (Data from: MacMahon B, Yen S, Trichopoulos D, Warren K, Nardi G. *N Engl J Med*, 1981; 304:630–633.)

A statistically significant difference, no matter how small the p_α, does not mean that the difference is clinically important. Certainly a statement like p <0.0001 is very impressive. If this p value emerges from a well-designed study, it does in fact convey a high degree of confidence that a difference really exists. But the p_α tells us nothing about the magnitude of that difference, or its clinical importance. In fact, entirely trivial differences may be highly statistically significant if a large enough number of subjects are studied.

Example—Two aminoglycoside antibiotics, gentamicin and tobramycin, are useful in many clinical situations because of their activity against a broad spectrum of bacteria. However, both can cause nephrotoxicity and ototoxicity. Preliminary evidence suggested that tobramycin was the less toxic of the two, and a study was done to examine this possibility.

Patients with suspected sepsis were randomly assigned to receive either gentamicin or tobramycin. Patients in the two groups were similar with respect to a variety of factors which might have predisposed them to renal disease.

The mean increase in serum creatinine was 0.4 mg per 100 ml for those given gentamicin and 0.1 mg per 100 ml for those given tobramycin. Nephrotoxicity (e.g., a rise of serum creatinine of 0.5 mg/100 ml or more) developed in 19 of 72 (26%) given gentamycin and 9 of 74 (12%) given tobramycin ($p < 0.025$).

Differences in toxicity were not large, and none of the patients was endangered by either drug. It was not reported whether peak levels of serum creatinine fell after the drugs were stopped. Therefore, although a statistically significant difference in nephrotoxicity was found between the two drugs, the clinical importance of the difference is not clear (3).

On the other hand, very unimpressive p_α's can result from studies showing strong treatment effects if there are few subjects in the study (see the following section).

For a given set of data, the p values obtained will depend on whether it is assumed from the outset that meaningful differences could only occur in one direction. For example, it might be generally believed that a relatively innocuous treatment could only help, and could not do harm. If we are prepared to make this assumption, then statistical tests can be conducted in such a way that a given difference favoring treatment is more likely to be statistically significant than if we are not. When the possibility of a difference in either direction is entertained, a *two-tailed* test of significance is used, whereas if we consider only differences in a particular direction, a *one-tailed* test is used. These terms come from the appearance of a curve describing the random variation in differences between treatments of equal value, where the two tails of the curve include statistically unlikely events favoring one or the other treatment (Figure 9.3).

There are differences of opinion about which approach—one- or two-tailed—is most appropriate in general, and for specific studies as well. Two-tailed tests are more conservative; they are less likely to conclude that a treatment works when it does not, but run a greater risk of missing a true difference favoring treatment. On the other hand, one-tailed tests assume one of the treatments is not worse, an assumption that is not necessarily correct.

Basic statistical tests, familiar to many readers, are used to estimate the probability of an α error. A summary of commonly used statistical tests, and the kinds of data for which they are used, is presented in Table 9.1. The validity of each test depends on certain assumptions about the data. If the data at hand do not satisfy these assumptions, the resulting p_α may be misleading. A discussion of how these statistical tests are derived and calculated, and of the assumptions upon which they rest, can be found in a number of excellent textbooks of biostatistics.

Statistics are also used to describe the degree of association between variables. Familiar expressions of association are Pearson's product moment correlation (r) for interval data and Spearman's rank correlation for ordinal data. Each of these statistics expresses in quantitative terms the extent to which the value of one variable is associated with the value of a second variable. Each has a corresponding statistical test, to assess whether the observed association is greater than might have arisen by chance alone.

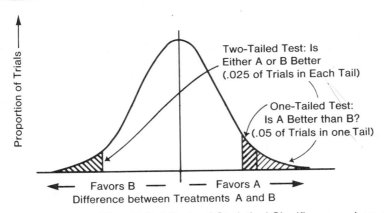

Figure 9.3.   One- and Two-Tailed Tests of Statistical Significance, where p_α = 0.05). A Larger Difference in Favor of Treatment A is Required for Statistical Significance if the Analysis is Done Assuming that Either A or B Might Be Better.

Table 9.1
Some Commonly Used Statistical Tests

Test	Statistic	Use
Chi-Square	χ^2	Comparing counts of discrete variables
Student's t-Test	t statistic	Comparing two means
Analysis of Variance	F-statistic	Comparing two or more means

CONCLUDING A TREATMENT DOES NOT WORK

Some trials come to the conclusion that a new treatment is no better than the old. There are some very influential examples: work showing that coronary artery bypass surgery does not prolong life in patients with chronic stable angina (except for those with left main coronary artery obstruction); early studies showing that antacids did not affect healing of duodenal ulcers; and the failure of insulin, as compared to diet alone, to prolong life in patients with mild diabetes mellitus.

The question arises: could results like these have occurred by chance alone? Could the findings of such trials have misrepresented the truth because these particular studies had the bad luck to turn out in relatively unlikely ways? The probability of this kind of error, the β or Type II error, is expressed as p_β.

Until recently, it has been unusual to find a careful consideration of p_β when the results of clinical trials were presented. Why have "negative trials" been subjected to the appropriate statistical testing so infrequently? For one thing, the mathematical basis of p_β is more difficult to conceptualize than p_α. Beta is relatively tough going for beginners. As a result, nearly all the space in introductory textbooks is devoted to p_α and usually only a few pages are given to p_β. Because most of us never get beyond introductory statistics, if that, we have very little exposure to the possibility of β error.

It may also be that β is neglected because we all simply prefer things that work. Negative results are unwelcome for most studies. If negative studies are reported at all, the authors may prefer to emphasize subgroups of subjects in which treatment differences are found, even if the differences are not statistically significant. Authors may also focus on reasons other than chance why true differences might have been missed.

Whatever the reason for not considering the probability of β error, it is the main question which should be asked when the results of a study indicate "no difference." Often the risk of β error is surprisingly large. In a recent survey of 71 published controlled trials showing no therapeutic benefit, 67 had a greater than 10% risk of missing a true therapeutic improvement of 25% (4). Fifty of the 71 trials had at least a 10% risk of missing a 50% improvement. The authors commented that "either these trials were almost uniformly undersized in the planning stage or the expected reduction in the end point percentage due to the treatment under consideration was very much in excess of a 50% reduction, and the reduction did not take place."

The probability that a trial will find a statistically significant difference when a difference really exists is called *power*. _sensitivity_

can be increased
by ↑ N

$$\text{Power} = 1 - p_\beta$$

Power and p_β are complementary ways of expressing the same concept. Power is analogous to the sensitivity of a diagnostic test. In fact, one speaks of a study being powerful if it has a high probability of calling different all those treatments that really are different.

HOW MANY SUBJECTS ARE ENOUGH?

Suppose you are reading about a clinical trial comparing a promising new therapy to the current form of treatment. You are aware that random variation can be the source of whatever differences are observed, and wonder if the number of subjects (sample size) in this study is sufficiently large as to make chance an unlikely explanation of what was found. How many subjects would be necessary to make an adequate comparison of the effects of the two treatments? The answer depends on four characteristics: the amount of variability among subjects, the difference in outcome between treatment groups, as well as p_α and p_β.

Variability *α sample size*

First, the appropriate sample size is determined by variability in outcome among the subjects of the study—that is, the extent to which subjects differ from each other with respect to prognosis. If there is relatively little difference in outcome from one subject to the next, then there will be less "noise" or unwanted variability introduced into the comparison between groups, and fewer subjects will be needed to be reasonably confident that the observed differences were not the result of chance. On the other hand, if the clinical course of subjects varies greatly—as it might, for example, for autoimmune diseases—then a larger number of patients would be necessary in order to distinguish true from chance differences. Unnecessary variability can be reduced by making careful measurements under standard conditions. However, some variability is a property of the disease and the patients under study, and cannot be reduced for the purposes of obtaining a sharper comparison.

may α 1/size

Difference *in magnitude outcome*

A second determinant of sample size is the magnitude of the difference to be detected. We are free to look for differences of any magnitude and, of course, we hope to be able to detect even very small differences. But more subjects are needed to detect small differences, everything else being equal. So it is best to ask only that there is a sufficient number of subjects to pick up the degree of improvement that would be clinically meaningful. On the other hand, if we are interested in detecting only very large differences between treated and control groups—i.e., strong treatment effects—then fewer subjects will be necessary.

Alpha Error *false (+) α important*

A third determinant of an adequate number of subjects is the risk of α error: falsely concluding that treatment is effective. The acceptable size for a risk of this kind is a value judgment. There are no theoretical limits as to how large or small that risk must be (short of 0 and 1). If one is prepared to accept the consequences of a large chance of falsely concluding the therapy is valuable, one can reach conclusions with relatively few subjects. On the other hand, if one wants to take only a small risk of being wrong in this way, a larger number of subjects will be required. As we discussed earlier, it is customary to set p_α at 0.05 (1 in 20) or sometimes 0.01.

Beta Error *false (−) α import.*

The chosen risk of a β error is the last determinant of sample size. This is also a judgment that can be freely made, and changed, to suit individual tastes. When p_β is considered, it is often set at 0.20 (a 20% chance of missing true differences).

Interrelationships

The relationships among these four variables are summarized in Table 9.2. The adequate number of subjects is related to the square of the four variables, rather than being related one to one. This means that for a change in the value of any one of them, N changes in geometric proportion. For example, to detect a treatment effect which is half as large, it would take about four times as many subjects.

The four variables in Table 9.2 can be traded off against each other. In general, for any given number of subjects there is a trade-off between α and β error. Everything else being equal, the more one is willing to accept one kind of error, the less it will be necessary to risk the other. Neither kind of error is inherently worse than the other. The consequences of using erroneous information depend on the clinical situation. When a better treatment is badly needed—for example, when the disease is very dangerous and no satisfactory alternative treatment is available—it would be reasonable to accept a relatively high risk of concluding a new treatment is effective when it really is not (large α error) in order to minimize the possibility of missing a valuable treatment (low β error). On the other hand, if the disease is less serious, alternative treatments are available, or the new treatment is expensive or dangerous, one might

Table 9.2
Determinants of Sample Size

N	varies as the square of	$\dfrac{V}{\Delta,\ p_\alpha,\ p_\beta}$

Where:

N = number of subjects
V = an expression of variability
Δ = difference in outcome between groups
p_α = risk of α (Type I) error
p_β = risk of β (Type II) error

want to minimize the risk of accepting the new treatment when it is not really effective (low α error), even at the expense of a relatively large chance of missing an effective treatment (large β error). It is of course possible to reduce both α and β error if the number of subjects is increased, variability decreased, or a larger treatment effect is sought.

For conventional levels of p_α and p_β, the effect of the strength of treatment on the number of subjects is illustrated by the following examples, one representing a situation in which a very large number of subjects was required, and the other in which a relatively small number of subjects was sufficient.

Example of large N—A trial was performed to compare the efficacy of two treatments for postmenopausal women with advanced breast cancer. Women were randomly assigned to receive either diethylstilbesterol or tamoxifen, and regression of tumor was used as an end point.

It would have been clinically important to detect differences in outcome as small as 10%. However, the authors estimated that to detect a 10% difference in regression probabilities (i.e., 30% versus 40% regression), with 80% power and p_α = 0.05 (one-tailed), about 280 patients would have been required in each treatment group. In fact, only 151 women could be entered into the study over a 3-year period, even though the study was conducted in a large referral center (The Mayo Clinic). This number of patients was large enough to detect a doubling in regression probabilities (i.e., 20% versus 40%) with a power of 0.74.

The authors had to settle for a smaller study than they would have preferred because the number of patients required to detect small but clinically important differences was unfeasibly large (5).

Example of Small N—To evaluate the efficacy of cimetidine in severe duodenal ulceration, 40 patients with active duodenal ulcers seen on endoscopy were randomly allocated to receive cimetidine 1 gram/day or placebo. After four weeks, a second endoscopy was performed by physicians who did not know which treatment had been given. Ulcer healing was observed in 17 of 20 patients receiving cimetidine and five of 20 patients receiving placebo. This difference was highly statistically significant (p < 0.0005) (6).

In this trial, the treatment effect was so powerful that relatively few subjects were needed to establish it.

These examples also illustrate that statistical power can be taken into account at two stages of clinical research: before data are collected, to assure that the objectives of the study can be met, and after the study is completed, to see if its conclusions are justified.

Until now, we have referred to the number of subjects needed for an adequately sensitive clinical trial, when each subject experiences an outcome of some sort. However, when outcomes for each patient are expressed as either/or events (e.g., death, recurrence of tumor, etc.) and not every patient experiences an event, power is more closely related to the number of events, not subjects. As Peto et al put it:

> In clinical trials of time to death (or of the time to some other particular "event"—relapse, metastasis, first thrombosis, stroke, recurrence, or time to death from a particular cause), the ability of the trial to distinguish between the merits of two treatments depends on how many patients die (or suffer a relevant event) rather than on the number of patients entered. A study of 100 patients, 50 of whom die, is about as sensitive as a study with 1000 patients, 50 of whom die (7).

Thus, more subjects must be entered in a trial if outcome events are relatively infrequent than if many of the subjects will experience an outcome event during the follow-up period.

For most of the therapeutic questions we encounter today, a surprisingly large number of subjects are required. The value of dramatic, powerful treatments—like insulin for diabetic ketoacidosis—could be established with a small number of subjects. But such treatments come along rarely, and many of them are already well established. We are left with diseases, many of them chronic, for which advances are usually modest, and come about through small increments. This places special importance on whether the size of clinical trials is adequate to distinguish real from chance effects.

Clinicians should develop some facility for estimating the power of published studies. Toward that end, Figure 9.4 shows the relationship between sample size and treatment difference for the situation in which outcome is dicotomous (alive or dead), $p_\alpha = 0.05$ and power is 50%. It is apparent from Figure 9.4 that studies involving fewer than 100 subjects have a rather poor chance of detecting statistically significant differences of even large treatment effects. A variety of journal articles and textbooks provide tables that make it possible to find any one of the variables, given the other three.

MULTIPLE COMPARISONS

The statistical conclusions of research have an aura of authority that defies challenge, particularly by non-experts. But as many skeptics have

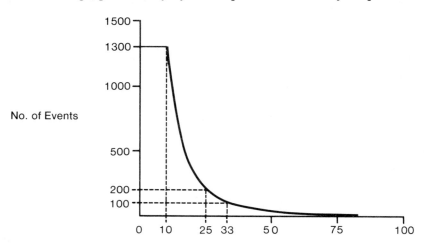

% Reduction in Events for Treated Group

Figure 9.4. The Difficulty Establishing Small Treatment Effects. The Approximate Number of Outcome Events Required to Have a 50–50 Chance ($P_\beta = 0.5$) of Finding a Statistically Significant Effect of Treatment ($p_\alpha < 0.05$), According to Degree of Benefit. For a controlled trial in which patients are randomized equally between two treatments. (From Peto R, Pike MC, Armitage P, Breslow NE, Cox DR, Howard SV, Mantel N, McPherson K, Peto J, Smith PG. *Br J Cancer*, 1976; 34:585–612.)

suspected, it is possible to "lie with statistics." What is more, lies are possible even if the research is well designed, the mathematics flawless, and the investigators' intentions beyond reproach.

Statistical conclusions can be misleading because the strength of statistical tests depends on the number of research questions considered in the study, and when those questions were asked. If many comparisons are made among the variables in a large set of data, the p value associated with each individual comparison is an underestimate of how often the result of that comparison, among the others, is likely to arise by chance. As implausible as it might seem, the interpretation of the p value from a single statistical test depends on the context in which it is done.

To understand how this might happen, consider the following example. Suppose a large study has been done in which there are multiple subgroups of patients, and many different outcomes. For example, it might be a clinical trial of the value of a treatment for coronary artery disease, where patients fall into several clinically meaningful groups (e.g., 1, 2, and 3-vessel disease, good and bad ventricular function, the presence or absence of arrhythmias, and various combinations of these) and several outcomes are considered (e.g., death, myocardial infarction, angina, etc.). Suppose also that there are no true associations between treatment and outcome for any of the subgroups and any of the outcomes. Finally, suppose that the effects of treatment are assessed separately for each subgroup and for each outcome—a process that involves a great many comparisons. As pointed out earlier in this chapter, at p = 0.05, one in 20 of these comparisons is likely to be statistically significant. If 40 comparisons are made, it could be expected that about two would be found statistically significant; if 100 comparisons are made, about five would be likely to emerge as significant; and so on. Because a great many comparisons have been made, there is a chance that a few will be found which are unusual enough, because of random variation, that they exceed the level of statistical significance even though no true associations between variables exist in nature. The more comparisons that are made, the more likely that one of them will be found statistically significant.

The situation we have just described is referred to as the *multiple comparisons* problem. Because of this problem, the strength of evidence from clinical research depends on how focused its questions were at the outset.

At one end of the spectrum, a study may be intended to assess the effect of one treatment on one outcome. In this case, an appropriate p value is a fair estimate of the role of chance. Such a study is called an *hypothesis testing* study because it can test hypothesis about the relationship between the treatment and the outcome.

At the other end of the spectrum, a study may either not specify a limited number of questions at the outset or may go beyond these questions to search the data for all possible associations. The unflattering name "data dredging" has been given to this process, although it may be undertaken to discover unanticipated relationships or to get the most out of a hard-won set of data. In this situation, there is a very real possibility that some statistically significant associations will be found by chance alone. Because of this problem, research involving multiple comparisons is best considered as a source of new hypotheses, not as a means of establishing that any one of them is true. Such studies are called *hypothesis generating*. Associations found after an exhaustive search of the data are at a relatively high risk of arising by chance alone, a risk much greater than their stated p value. The following is an example of hypothesis-generating research.

Example—A study was done to explore whether there were adverse health effects on people living near a chemical dump. It was not known at the outset just what those effects might be. Residents were interviewed and examined, and information on a total of 180 different variables was obtained. The frequency with which these variables were reported among those exposed to the chemical dump was compared to similar information from a national survey. Nine responses (5%) were significantly more common at the 0.025 level. They included hiatus hernia, frequent cough, use of skin medicines, etc.—none of which seemed plausibly related to chemicals. It was concluded that the study provided no evidence in favor of toxic effects (8).

Unfortunately, when the results of research are presented, it is not always possible to know how many comparisons were really made. Often interesting findings are selected from a larger number of uninteresting ones. This process of deciding what is and is not important about a mass of data can introduce considerable distortion of reality.

How can the statistical effects of multiple comparisons be taken into account when interpreting research? Although a variety of ways of adjusting p_α have been proposed, for the present the best advice is to be aware of the problem and to be cautious about accepting conclusions of studies where multiple comparisons were made. As one statistician put it:

" . . . if you dredge the data sufficiently deep and sufficiently often, you will find something odd. Many of these bizarre findings will be due to chance. I do not imply that data dredging is not an occupation for honorable persons, but rather that discoveries that were not initially postulated as among the major objectives of the trial should be treated with extreme caution. Statistical theory may in due course show us how to allow for such incidental findings. At present, I think the best attitude to adopt is caution, coupled with an attempt to confirm or refute the findings by further studies" (9).

SUMMARY

Clinical information is based on observations made on samples of patients. Yet even unbiased samples may misrepresent events in a larger population of such patients, because of the effects of random variation among its members.

Inferential statistics are used to estimate the role of random variation in clinical observations. When two treatments are compared, there are two ways in which the conclusions of the trial can be wrong: the treatments may be no different and it is concluded one is better; or one treatment may be better and it is concluded there is no difference. The probabilities that these errors will occur in a given situation are given by p_α and p_β, respectively.

The power of a statistical test $(1 - p_\beta)$ is the probability of finding a statistically significant difference when a difference really exists. Statistical power is related to the number of subjects (events) in the trial, size of the treatment effect, variability in outcome, and p_α. Everything else being equal, power can be increased by increasing the number of subjects in a trial, but that is not always feasible.

Reported p values may underestimate the role of chance if a great many comparisons are made on a given set of data. In such situations, statistical tests of significance should be interpreted with caution.

Suggested Readings

Feinstein AR. Clinical Biostatistics. Section 4. Mathematical Mistiques and Statistical Strategies. St. Louis: C.V. Mosby Co., 1977.

Swinscow, TDV. Statistics at Square One. London: British Medical Association, 1978.

Colton T. Statistics in Medicine. Boston: Little, Brown and Co. 1974.

Rothman KHJ. A show of confidence. *N Engl J Med*, 1978; 299:1362–1363.

Berwick DM. Experimental power: the other side of the coin. *Pediatrics*, 1980; 65:1043–1045.

Freiman JA, Chalmers TC, Smith H, Kuebler RR. The importance of beta, the type II error and sample size in the design and interpretation of the randomized control trial. *N Engl J Med*, 1978; 299:690–694.

Tukey JW. Some thoughts on clinical trials, especially problems of multiplicity. *Science*, 1977; 198:679–684.

References

1. Schor S. The mystic statistic. Aids to the Understanding of Statistical Methods and Terms in Medicine. Reprinted with permission from the *Journal of the American Medical Association*.
2. MacMahon B, Yen S, Trichopoulos D, Warren K, Nardi G. Coffee and cancer of the pancreas. *N Engl J Med* 1981; 304:630–633.
3. Smith CR, Lipsky JJ, Laskin OL, Hellmann DB, Mellits ED, Longstreth J, Lietman PS. Double-blind comparison of the nephrotoxicity and auditory toxicity of gentamicin and tobramycin. *N Engl J Med*, 1980; 302:1106–1109.
4. Freiman JA, Chalmers TC, Smith H, Kuebler RR. The importance of beta type II error and sample size in the design and interpretation of the randomized control trial. *N Engl Med*, 1978; 299:690–694.
5. Ingle JN, Ahmann DL, Green SJ, Edmonson JH, Bisel HF, Kvols LK, Nichols WC, Creagan ET, Hahn RG, Rubin J, Frytak S. Randomized clinical trial of diethylstilbesterol versus tamoxifen in postmenopausal women with advanced breast cancer. *N Engl J Med* 1981; 304:16–21.
6. Gray GR, McKenzie I, Smith IS, Crean GP, Gillespie G. Oral cimetidine in severe duodenal ulceration. A double-blind controlled trial. *Lancet*, 1977; 1:4–7.
7. Peto R, Pike MC, Armitage P, Breslow NE, Cox DR, Howard SV, Mantel N, McPherson K, Peto J, Smith PG. Design and analysis of randomized clinical trials requiring prolonged observation of each patient. I. Introduction and design. *Br J Cancer*, 1976; 34:585–612.
8. Center for Disease Control. Morbidity Study at a Chemical Dump. *Morbid Mortal Report*, 1981; 30:294–295.
9. Armitage P. Importance of prognostic factors in the analysis of data from clinical trials. *Controlled Clin Trials*, 1981; 1:347–353.

chapter

10

Rare Disease

It has been estimated that 90% of medical school curriculum time considers 10% of mankind's morbidity. This estimate has been used to derogate the emphasis placed by academic centers on rare diseases. But it also highlights an inescapable fact—most diseases are, thankfully, not common. For example, we read repeatedly about the current epidemic of bronchogenic carcinoma, the "plague of the 20th century." Whereas the bubonic plague killed in a matter of months as many as 60–70% of the residents of afflicted cities and villages in 14th century Europe, bronchogenic carcinoma will kill approximately 3–4% of older men over a 10-year period. Although certainly a tragic and largely preventable disease, this "common" killer will be diagnosed only once a year or less by the average primary care physician. To put this frequency into the perspective of a cohort study, 3000 older men must be followed for at least 10 years in order to obtain information about 100 cases.

What about the prevalence of the common chronic diseases? After all, prevalence provides a better estimate of the physician's case load than incidence. Asthma, generally considered a relatively common disease, was reported by 3% of a random sample of Americans. However, the large majority of these people (80% or more) suffered no disability related to their asthma and 30% did not visit a physician for any reason during a one-year period (1). Based on these figures, it has been estimated that the identification of 200 asthmatics under age 55 would require a survey of 2300 households or the review of 10,700 medical records from primary care practices (2).

The uncommonness of most diseases has led to the development of massive, often collaborative multi-center studies when information about incidence or the effect of treatment on outcomes is needed. However, the difficulties attending the acquisition of large numbers of patients with a given condition, illustrated previously, have forced investigators and clinicians to confine their observations on many diseases to relatively small numbers of people. The question is whether studies of small numbers of patients are useful to the practitioner facing problems of diagnosis, prognosis, cause, or treatment, given all the pitfalls described in the preceding chapters. Or, to turn the question around a little, under what circumstances can observations on small numbers of patients prove useful?

THE CASE REPORT

Case reports are detailed presentations of a single case or a handful of cases. They represent an important way in which unusual diseases or unusual presentations of disease are brought to the attention of the medical community. A systematic review of the original articles published in the *Journal of the American Medical Association, The Lancet,* and *the New England Journal of Medicine* in the years 1946, 1956, 1966, and 1976 revealed that 38% of all research reports in these prestigious journals studied 10 or fewer subjects and 13% discussed a single case (3). Reports of rare events, therefore, are not rare.

Case reports serve several different purposes which must be distinguished before trying to decide their clinical utility.

First, case reports are virtually our only means of surveillance for rare events. Therefore, they are a rich source of ideas (hypotheses) about disease frequency, risk, prognosis, and treatment. Case reports rarely can be used to test these hypotheses. But they do place issues before the medical community, and often trigger more decisive studies of disease. Some conditions which were first recognized through case reports include birth defects from thalidomide, the fetal alcohol syndrome, and some of the legionella infections.

Case reports also serve to elucidate the mechanisms of disease and treatment by reporting highly detailed and methodologically sophisticated clinical and laboratory studies of a patient or small group of patients. In this instance, the complexity, cost, and the often experimental nature of the investigations limit their application to small numbers of subjects. Such highly detailed studies have contributed a great deal to our understanding of the genetic, metabolic, and physiologic basis of a large number of human diseases. These studies represent the bridge between laboratory research and clinical research and have a well-established place in the annals of medical progress.

The following is an example of how a report of a single case can reveal a great deal about the mechanism of a disease.

Example—The anesthetic halothane has been suspected of causing hepatitis. However, because the frequency of hepatitis after exposure to halothane is low, and there are many other causes of hepatitis after surgery, "halothane hepatitis" has remained controversial.

Experience with a single individual helped to clarify the problem. An anesthetist was found to have recurrent hepatitis, leading to cirrhosis. Attacks of hepatitis regularly recurred within hours of his return to work. When he was exposed to small doses of halothane, his hepatitis recurred and was well documented by clinical observations, biochemical tests and liver histology.

Because of this unusual case, it is clear that halothane can cause hepatitis. But the case report provides no information on how often this occurs (4).

Another use of the case report is to present unusual manifestations of disease. Sometimes this can become the medical version of Ripley's *Believe It or Not*, an informal compendium of medical oddities where the interest lies in the sheer unbelievability of the case. The larger the lesion and the more outrageous the foreign body or its location, the more likely a case report is to find its way into the literature. Oddities that are simply bizarre aberrancies from the usual course of events may titillate but reveal little of clinical importance.

Some so-called oddities are, however, the result of a fresher, more insightful look at a problem and prove to be the first evidence of a subsequently useful finding. The problem for the reader is how to distinguish between the freak and the fresh insight. There are no rules of which we are aware. When all else fails, one can only rely on common sense and a well-developed sense of skepticism.

Because case reports involve a small and highly selected group of patients, they are particularly susceptible to bias. For example, case reports of successful therapy may be misleading because journals are unlikely to receive or publish case reports of unsuccessful therapy. A recent study examined the effectiveness of postmortem Caesarean section in an attempt to save the baby, as described in 105 instances found in 63 case reports, and 72 instances reported from a single community-based study (5). The contrast in findings was striking; whereas 57% of the infants described in case reports survived, only 15% of infants in the community-based study survived. The obvious explanation rests with the bias of authors to write up and journal editors to accept for publication the unusual: in this example, those cases with an unusually happy ending. At the other extreme, disasters written up in case reports often prove, on more systematic study of larger populations, to be rare phenomena.

Perhaps the wisest stance to take when reviewing a case report is to use it as a signal to look for further evidence of the described phenomenon in the literature or among your patients. With very few exceptions, case reports should not serve as the basis for altering clinical practice because of their inherent biases and their inability to estimate the frequency of the described occurrence or the role of chance.

THE CASE SERIES

A *case series* is a prevalence survey of a group of individuals with a particular disease, performed at a single point in time. It is a particularly common way of delineating the clinical picture of a rare disease, and serves this purpose well—but with some important limitations.

First, case series describe, in quantitative terms, the clinical manifestations of disease, both purported causes and effects, at one point in time. They must be distinguished, therefore, from prognostic studies or uncontrolled trials of treatment where a cohort of patients with a disease is followed over time looking for the outcomes of the disease. Case series do not have a time dimension and that restricts their value as a means of studying cause-effect relationships.

Case series also suffer from the absence of a comparison group. As a result, it is difficult to put observed associations in context.

Example—In one typical case series, the authors described a new association between erythroleukemia and rheumatic complaints. The association was inferred from the fact that 30% of their patients with erythroleukemia had unexplained pain. Also, when a small subgroup of patients was tested, immunological abnormalities were "numerous" (0–67% of patients for different tests).

The authors concluded that "the clinical complex described should be searched for in all cases of erythroleukemia." However, whether this is, in fact, an unusually high prevalence of rheumatic pain and immunologic abnormalities can only be determined by comparison with other groups of very sick patients referred to a world renowned cancer treatment center and receiving blood transfusions, cytotoxic drugs, and other treatments. The absence of this comparison forces the reader to rely exclusively on the authors' judgment as to whether the prevalence of rheumatic complaints and immunologic abnormalities is high enough to be meaningful (6).

However, case series describe a larger number of patients than do case reports. It is possible, therefore, to assess the role of chance when interpreting the internal validity of case series. At the minimum, about 10 cases are required to assess statistical significance because with fewer cases, statistical tests for estimating the role of chance are not powerful enough to detect even very large differences. For example, when one flips a coin seven times, the only statistically significant results are seven heads or seven tails.

THE CASE CONTROL STUDY

Whether a given prevalence is high enough or low enough to be important can be understood better if the same observations are made on another group, or several groups, of controls, which are comparable. Studies which compare the frequency of clinical findings or causal factors in a group of cases and a group of controls have been termed *case control studies*. Another name for this kind of study design is *retrospective*.

A distinguishing feature of the case control design, which contributes to its fallibility, is that cases possess the outcome of interest at the time that the clinical findings or causal factors are measured. For example, a case control study of the influence of bacteriuria in young girls on renal status in adulthood would compare the frequency of past bacteriuria in a group of women with renal disease (the cases) and a group of women with normal kidneys (the controls). The outcome of interest, renal disease, has already occurred. This research strategy must be contrasted with a deceptively similar but fundamentally different approach in which a group of girls with bacteriuria and a group of girls with sterile urine cultures are identified and then examined over time for the development of renal disease. Such a study is simply a variation of the usual cohort design described in Chapter 6.

Figure 10.1 illustrates the differences between cohort and case control

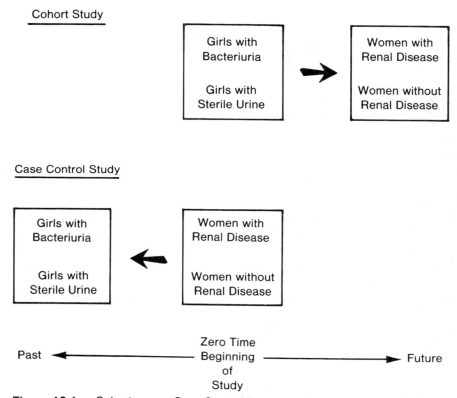

Figure 10.1.   Cohort versus Case Control Approaches to Studying the Possible Effect of Childhood Bacteriuria on Renal Disease in Adult Women.

approaches. In essence, a case control study is a backward look at two or more groups of patients, a group of cases with the outcome of interest and one or more groups of controls without the outcome of interest.

Advantages of Case Control Studies

The case control design has emerged as the most important method used to study rare diseases. What are its advantages?

First, the investigators can identify cases unconstrained by the natural frequency of disease, and yet can still make a comparison. Cohort studies are quite inefficient for this purpose. For example, in order to gather information about the risk of estrogen use in 100 women with endometrial cancer, one would have to follow a cohort of 10,000 postmenopausal women for about 10 years. Obviously, the expense and logistic difficulties of such a study would usually render it unrealistic. In contrast, it has been relatively inexpensive and easy to assemble a hundred or more cases from hospitals and other treatment facilities, find similar groups of women without the disease and compare frequencies of past estrogen use. In this way, several hundred women can be interviewed in a matter of weeks or months and an answer can be obtained at a fraction of the cost of a cohort study.

A second advantage of the case control study in exploring the effect of causal or prognostic factors relates to the concept of latency or the necessity for a period of time to elapse between exposure to a factor and the expression of its pathologic effects. For example, it has been estimated that 15 or more years may pass before the carcinogenicity of various chemicals becomes manifest. It would require an extremely patient investigator and scientific community to wait for 15 years to see if a suspected risk to health can be confirmed.

Because of their ability to address important questions rapidly and efficiently, case control studies play an increasingly important role in the medical literature. According to recent surveys of leading medical journals, case control studies now comprise 5–10% of all original articles and 30–40% of all epidemiologic articles (7). Their quickness and cheapness justify this popularity as long as their results are valid, and here is the fly in the ointment.

In general, case control studies are particularly prone to biased results. Walking through the steps involved in such a study, and the necessarily tough decisions facing the investigators, should clarify the unique vulnerabilities to bias that this approach entails.

Cohort Versus Case Control

A cohort study designed to see if estrogen therapy is a risk factor for endometrial cancer would begin by identifying several thousand postmenopausal women, screening them for endometrial cancer and removing from the cohort those with evidence of the disease (Figure 10.2). The remaining women would be interviewed about their current use of drugs including estrogens; the interviews could, of course, be confirmed by examining the patients' current medications, pharmacy records and physicians' records. Detailed information about the chemical composition, dose, timing of doses, and duration of therapy would be obtained, checked, and recorded. The women would be periodically and uniformly re-examined for endometrial cancer and estrogen use; any woman not appearing for the regular examination would be vigorously pursued so as to maintain surveillance and to gather information about her current status. These examinations would continue until a sufficient number of new cases of endometrial cancer had been observed to allow a firm conclusion about the risk of estrogen use.

As described in Chapter 6, the researchers would be able to measure directly the risk or incidence of endometrial cancer in estrogen users and non-users and compute a relative risk of estrogen use by dividing the incidence in users by the incidence in non-users. If relative risk exceeded one, was unlikely to exceed one simply by chance alone (i.e., the p value was very low, <0.05) and estrogen users and non-users did not differ substantially with regard to other risk factors for endometrial cancer (e.g., obesity and nulliparity), then it would be reasonable to accept that estrogen use is a risk factor for endometrial cancer. It would still be necessary to decide whether the association is causal, a decision which will be discussed further in Chapter 11.

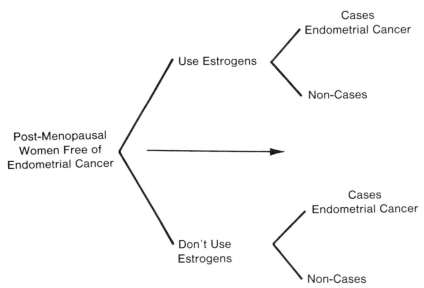

Figure 10.2.   Cohort Study of the Risk of Estrogens for Endometrial Cancer.

A case control study of the same question (Figure 10.3) provides a striking contrast to the hypothetical cohort study described above. First, the researchers must find a group of women suffering from endometrial cancer. For obvious reasons, they would look in hospitals or other cancer treatment centers where many such cases are gathered. The cases, therefore, would not include those who have rapidly succumbed to their disease and would include only women in whom the diagnosis had been made in the course of usual medical care. For example asymptomatic disease would be far less frequent in the latter situation.

Once the cases are assembled and the diagnosis confirmed, a comparison or control group must be selected. Before making this decision, the investigators must pause to consider the purpose of the study. They want to ascertain whether women with endometrial cancer were more likely to

have received estrogen therapy in the past than a similar group of women
fortunate enough to have been spared the disease.

What is meant by similar? Similarity in the cohort study meant
membership in the same cohort, for example, postmenopausal women
residing in a given community or attending the same clinic(s). Is there a
natural cohort from which a group of cases receiving care at a given
hospital can emerge? Because of referral practices, cases assembled at
hospitals and other treatment centers usually reside in many communi-
ties, receive their care from many physicians, and belong to no common
group before becoming ill. Therefore, there is no obviously similar group
of women without endometrial cancer and one must be created. This is
generally done by finding women who are in the hospital for reasons
other than endometrial cancer and/or women residing in the same

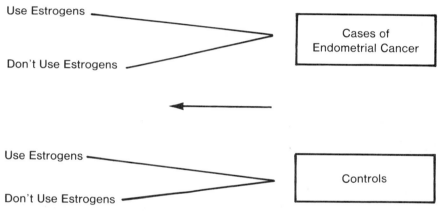

Figure 10.3.   Case-Control Study of the Risk of Estrogens for Endometrial
Cancer.

neighborhoods as the cases. In this way, a group of women is assembled
who are hopefully similar to cases with respect to factors that might
determine risk for endometrial cancer, other than estrogens.

Once the cases and controls have been selected and their consent
obtained, the next step is to measure the exposure or characteristic of
interest. To examine the possible risk of estrogen therapy, each woman's
drug-taking history must be reconstructed for both cases and controls.
As opposed to the cohort study, this will rely on memory and the
availability and completeness of medical records. It is the past, not the
present, which is important and therein lies a potential for bias in case
control studies. As every student of history knows, it is difficult not to
interpret the past in the light of one's present condition. For patients,
this is particularly so when the present includes a disease as serious as
cancer. Investigators attempt to avoid bias by using carefully defined
criteria to decide which of the cases and controls received prior estrogen
therapy.

Case Control versus Prevalence Survey

A prevalence survey examining the possible risk of estrogens for endometrial cancer would begin and end as the cohort study began—by a single examination of a large population of postmenopausal women for endometrial cancer and estrogen use. In the prevalence survey approach, the cases would include all those found in the population during the survey and the non-cases would include all of the large number of women free of the disease. Unlike the case control study outlined previously, we can be certain that both cases and non-cases were members of the same population group. Like the case control study, however, the estrogen exposure history has to be reconstructed from interviews and medical records.

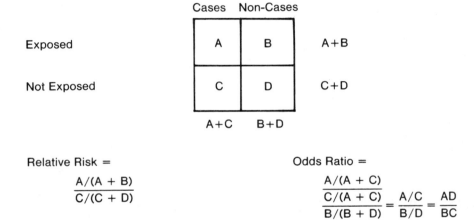

Figure 10.4. 2 × 2 Table Showing How Association Between an Exposure and Disease is Calculated for Cohort and Case Control Studies.

The Odds Ratio

How do we decide whether there is an increased risk? Figure 10.4 shows the calculation of risk for cohort and case control studies.

In a cohort study, the susceptible population is divided into two groups—exposed (A+B) and unexposed (C+D)—at the outset. Cases of endometrial cancer emerge naturally over time in the exposed group (*A*) and the unexposed group (*C*). This provides us with appropriate numerators and denominators to calculate the incidences of endometrial cancer in the exposed (A/A + B) and unexposed (C/C + D) cohorts. It is also possible to calculate the relative risk.

$$\text{Relative Risk} = \frac{\text{Incidence of Disease in the Exposed}}{\text{Incidence of Disease in the Unexposed}} = \frac{A/A + B}{C/C + D}$$

Case control studies, on the other hand, begin with the selection of a group of cases (A + C) and another group of controls (B + D). Disease rates are meaningless, because these groups are determined not by nature, but by the investigators' selection criteria. Therefore, aň incidence (or, for that matter, a prevalence) rate of disease among those exposed to estrogen and those not exposed cannot be computed. Consequently, it is not possible to obtain relative risk by dividing incidence among users by incidence among non-users. What does have meaning, however, are the relative frequencies of women exposed to estrogens among the cases and controls.

It is possible to obtain an estimate of relative risk in another way. In fact, the rapid increase in the use of the case control design was due, in part, to the contributions of biostatisticians and epidemiologists who demonstrated that one approach for comparing the frequency of exposure among cases and controls provided a measure of risk which is conceptually and mathematically similar to the relative risk. This is the *odds ratio*, defined as the odds that a case is exposed

$$\left(\frac{A/A+C}{C/A+C}\right)$$

divided by the odds that a control is exposed

$$\left(\frac{B/B+D}{D/B+D}\right)$$

The odds ratio simplifies to

$$\frac{A/C}{B/D} \text{ or } \frac{A\ D}{B\ C}$$

which, as is seen in Figure 10.4, results from multiplying diagonally across the table and then dividing these cross-products.

Note that if the frequency of exposure is higher among cases, the odds ratio will exceed one, indicating risk. Conversely, if the frequency of exposure is lower among cases, the odds ratio will be less than one, indicating protection. Thus, the stronger the association between the exposure and disease, the higher the odds ratio. The meaning of the odds ratio, therefore, is analogous to the relative risk obtained in cohort studies. The similarity of the information conveyed by the odds ratio and the relative risk have led most investigators to report odds ratios as "relative risk estimates" or even "relative risks." Whether this assumption is fully justified is still subject to dispute; however, the odds ratio has proven to be a useful measure of the effect of an exposure on the outcome.

In a prevalence survey, disease rates can be computed which are, of course, prevalences, not incidences. Prevalence rates in the exposed and unexposed can be divided to produce a ratio which closely resembles a relative risk. Recalling that prevalence roughly equals incidence times duration, a relative risk computed from prevalence rates will approximately equal that computed from incidence rates if the duration of the disease is the same for the exposed and unexposed. However, often this is not the case. For example, continued smoking increases the rapidity of death in patients with lung cancer. This would tend to reduce the prevalence of lung cancer among smokers relative to non-smokers, making the relative risk of smoking seem lower than it actually is. For this reason, many epidemiologists prefer to use the odds ratio to estimate risk in prevalence surveys.

Table 10.1 summarizes the essential characteristics of the cohort, case control and prevalence research designs and illustrates their differences. As will be discussed later, it is these differences which make the case control study particularly susceptible to bias.

BIAS IN CASE CONTROL STUDIES

Bias in Selecting Groups

Although the word experimental is generally used by epidemiologists to refer to clinical trials, there are elements of experimental manipulation in case control studies as well. In case control research, the investigators manipulate the comparison groups rather than the exposure or treatment, whereas nature determines who becomes a case and who is fortunate enough to remain a non-case or control in a cohort or prevalence study. This element of manipulation is a necessary evil because if the investigator cannot achieve comparability of cases and controls, the findings will be dismissed.

Cases and controls are comparable if they were equally likely to have been exposed to the factor of interest under the assumption that the exposure is unrelated to the disease. In other words, to be comparable, cases and controls must seem to have had an equal chance of being exposed. For example, the opportunity to have received postmenopausal estrogens would presumably be greater among women who have received regular medical care and perhaps still greater among women who have received regular gynecologic care; thus, comparability as defined previously would be more acceptable if both cases and controls had similar medical care experiences. But how similar should they be? If one insists that cases and controls have the same doctor, the study may be nullified if that doctor systematically either prescribes or does not prescribe estrogens to all postmenopausal patients.

Therefore, ensuring comparability between cases and controls requires the careful consideration of the circumstances under which an individual becomes exposed. To return to an example mentioned in Chapter 1:

Example—In the first case control study reporting a positive association between reserpine and breast cancer, hospitalized women with cardiovascular diagnoses were excluded from the control group. Because hypertension is one of the main reasons for prescribing reserpine, and hypertension is likely to be common among patients with cardiovascular diagnoses, this exclusion probably removed reserpine takers from the control group. This would bias the results in favor of the conclusion that reserpine is associated with breast cancer. In the context of Figure 10.4, the exclusion of patients with cardiovascular diagnoses from the controls would reduce the B cell of the table which would reduce the denominator of the odds ratio AD/BC (8).

Strategies to Obtain Comparable Cases and Controls

Suffice it to say that the selection of a comparable control group is a difficult task. Simple rules prove inadequate because the decisions depend upon the particular exposure under study and the source and nature of

Table 10.1
Summary of Characteristics of Cohort, Case Control, and Prevalence Designs

Cohort	Case Control	Prevalence
1. Begins with a defined population at risk	Population at risk generally undefined	Begins with a defined population
2. Cases not selected but ascertained by continuous surveillance (presumably all cases)	Cases selected by investigator from an available pool of patients	Cases not selected but ascertained by a single examination of the population
3. Comparison group (i.e., non-cases) not selected— evolve naturally	Controls selected by investigator to resemble cases	Non-cases include those free of disease at the single examination
4. Exposure measured before the development of disease	Exposure measured, reconstructed, or recollected after development of disease	Exposure measured, reconstructed, or recollected after development of disease
5. Risk or incidence of disease and relative risk measured directly	Risk or incidence of disease cannot be measured directly: relative risk of exposure can be estimated by the odds ratio	Risk or incidence of disease cannot be measured directly: relative risk of exposure can be estimated by the odds ratio

the cases. Two strategies are now commonly used in an effort to achieve comparability.

First, cases can be *matched* with controls so that for each case one or more controls are selected who possess characteristics in common with the case. Researchers commonly match for age, race, and sex because these are frequently related to disease. But matching often extends beyond these demographic characteristics when other factors are known to be important.

If performed properly, matching maximizes the information obtainable from a set of cases and controls because this reduces differences between groups in determinants of disease other than the one being considered, and thereby allows for a more powerful (sensitive) test of association. But matching carries a risk. If the investigator happens to match on a factor which is itself related to exposure there is an increased chance that the matched case and control will have the same history of exposure. For example, if cases and controls were matched for hot flashes, which are commonly treated with estrogens, it would increase the likelihood that the two groups would have similar exposure to estrogens. This process, called over-matching, can result in a falsely low estimate of relative risk.

The second strategy is more straightforward and probably more valuable: choosing more than one control group. Because of the difficulties attending the selection of a truly comparable control group, a systematic error in the odds ratio may arise. A way to guard against this possibility is to choose more than one control group, particularly if they are drawn from different sources. One approach used when cases are drawn from a hospital is to choose one control group from other patients in the same hospital and a second control group from the neighborhoods of the cases. If similar odds ratios are obtained using different control groups, this is evidence against bias because it is unlikely that bias would affect otherwise dissimilar groups to the same extent. If the estimates of relative risks are different, that is a signal that one or both are biased, and an opportunity exists to investigate where the bias lies.

Example—In a recent case control study of estrogen and endometrial cancer, cases were identified from a single teaching hospital. Two control groups were selected: one from among gynecologic admissions to the same hospital and the second from a random sample of women living in the area served by the hospital.

Table 10.2 shows the distribution of various characteristics, including estrogen use, among these three groups. Note that the presence of other diseases such as hypertension, diabetes, or gallbladder disease was much more common among the two hospital groups, presumably reflecting the various forces that lead to hospitalization. Despite these differences, the two control groups reported much less long-term estrogen use than did the cases, and yielded very similar odds ratios (4.1 and 3.6).

The authors concluded that "this consistency of results with two very different comparison groups suggests that neither is significantly biased and that the results . . . are reasonably accurate" (9).

Bias in Measuring the Exposure

Even if selection bias can be avoided, the investigator then faces the problems associated with validly measuring exposure after the disease or outcome has occurred—that is, avoiding measurement bias. Three kinds of measurement bias can occur.

1. The presence of the outcome directly affects the exposure.
2. The presence of the outcome affects the subject's recollection of the exposure.
3. The presence of the outcome affects the measurement or recording of the exposure.

We will illustrate these, again using the example of estrogen and endo-metrial cancer.

First, it has been postulated that because endometrial cancer most commonly presents to physicians as postmenopausal vaginal bleeding, and estrogens are sometimes prescribed as treatment for postmenopausal bleeding, this therapeutic use of estrogens accounts for their association with endometrial cancer. Although this sequence of events has proven to be extremely rare, it represents one way in which the presence of an outcome can lead to exposure rather than vice versa.

Second, people with a disease may recall exposure differently from those without the disease. With all the publicity surrounding the possible risks of estrogen use, it is entirely possible that victims of endometrial cancer would remember their previous drug histories more accurately than non-victims, or even overestimate their estrogen use. The influence of disease on memory is illustrated by a study of the possible familial aggregation of rheumatoid arthritis (10). As shown in Table 10.3, patients

Table 10.2

Characteristics of Cases and Two Control Groups. A Case Control Study of Estrogen Exposure and Endometrial Cancer*

Characteristic	Cases	Gynecology Controls	Community Controls
No. of Subjects	186	153	236
Mean Age	60	60	55
% Nulliparous	27	14	16
% Obese	52	40	31
% Hypertensive	51	48	34
% Diabetic	19	17	7
% Gallbladder Disease	18	26	12
% Long-term (3.5 yr) Estro-gen Use	20	3	7

* Adapted from: Hulka BS, Fowler WC Jr, Kaufman DG, Greenberg BG, Hogue CJR, Berger GS, Pulliam CC. *Am J Obstet Gynecol* 1980; 137:92–101.

with rheumatoid arthritis were more likely to give a family history of rheumatoid arthritis than were controls. However, this association was not present when family histories given by the unaffected siblings of the rheumatoid arthritis cases were compared with those of controls. As we are all well aware, it is natural for sick people to seek explanations for their misfortunes; and backward research, as in case control or prevalence studies provides an opportunity for doing so.

Critical readers should look for two protections against biased remem-bering. First, there should be alternative sources of the same information, whether written documents such as medical or other records or interviews with relatives or other knowledgable individuals. Second, the specific purpose of the study should be concealed from the study subjects. It would be unethical not to inform subjects of the general nature of the study question. But to provide detailed information to subjects about the specific hypotheses could so bias the resulting information obtained as to commit another breach of ethics—involving subjects in a worthless research project.

The third problem, where the presence of the outcome influences the way in which the exposure is measured or recorded should be understandable by all past and present students of physical diagnosis. If a gynecology resident admitting a woman with endometrial cancer to the hospital is

Table 10.3

Effect of Outcome on Measurement of Exposure. Reported Family History of Rheumatoid Arthritis According to Whether or Not The Reporter Has the Disease*

Arthritis	Family History of Arthritis		
	Controls (%)	Rheumatoid Arthritis (RA) Patients (%)	Siblings of RA Patients (%)
Neither Parent	55	27	50
One Parent	37	58	42
Both Parents	8	15	8

* Adapted from: Sackett DL. *J Chron Dis*, 1979; 32:51–63; and Schull WJ and Cobb S. *J Chron Dis*, 1969; 22:217–222.

Table 10.4

Controversial Topics—Case Control Results*

	Support	Do Not Support
TB Protects Against Cancer	1	1
Lactation Protects Against Breast Cancer	2	4
Circumcision Protects Against Cervical Cancer	2	6
Prenatal Irradiation Causes Leukemia	7	3
Allergy Protects Against Malignancy	3	3
Appendectomy Causes Malignancy	3	4
Early Menarche Causes Breast Cancer	3	3
Herpes Virus Causes Cervical Cancer	1	1
Birth Control Pills Protect Against Benign Breast Disease	4	2
Coffee Causes Bladder Cancer	3	2
Tonsillectomy Causes Hodgkin's Disease	2	3
Coffee Causes Coronary Heart Disease	2	2
Reserpine Causes Breast Cancer	3	8
Estrogens Cause Endometrial Cancer	9	2

* Adapted from: Horwitz RI, Feinstein AR. *Am J Med*, 1979; 66:556–564.

aware of a possible link between estrogen use and endometrial cancer one could expect the resident to question the patient more intensely about previous hormone use and to record the information more carefully. Interviewers who are aware of a possible relationship between exposure and disease and also the outcome status of the interviewee would be remarkable indeed if they conducted identical interviews for cases and controls. The protections against these sources of bias are the same as those mentioned above: multiple sources of information and blinding the data gatherers (i.e., keeping them in the dark as to the hypothesis under study).

Role in Medical Controversy

Because of their susceptibility to bias, case control studies of the same question have all too often yielded conflicting results (11). Table 10.4 illustrates the "contribution" of this study design to several important scientific controversies over the past few decades. In fairness, several of these have been resolved by more carefully designed and executed case control studies which paid greater attention to possible sources of bias.

SUMMARY

Rare diseases, because they occur so infrequently, must often be studied using less than optimal research designs. Case reports are studies of just a few patients (e.g., ≤ 10). They have been a useful means of surveillance for rare disease, describing rare presentations of disease, as well as understanding the mechanisms of disease. However, case reports are of little help in characterizing the frequency of disease, and they are particularly prone to bias and chance. Case series describe patients at a single point in time. They suffer from the absence of a reference group with which to compare the experience of the cases.

In case control studies, a group of cases is compared with a similar group of non-cases (controls). This approach has seen increasing use in the study of rare disease. Its advantage resides in the ability to assemble cases from treatment centers as opposed to finding them or waiting for them to develop in a defined population at risk. Thus, case control studies are much less expensive and much quicker to perform than cohort studies. It is not possible to compute incidences from case control studies nor can relative risk be obtained directly. However, relative risk can be estimated by the odds ratio. The disadvantages of the case-control design all relate to its considerable susceptibility to bias. Two characteristics of case control research create this problem: first, the groups to be compared are selected by the researcher and are not constituted naturally; second, the exposure is measured after the disease has already occurred.

Given the vulnerability of case control studies to bias, what place do they have in clinical epidemiologic research? To some, case control studies are unscientific, illogical, and a curse. To others, they are viewed as the essential first step in studying most medically important questions. There is nearly universal agreement, however, that cohort studies provide the strongest, most valid evidence and, if feasible, are the design of choice. But with appropriate attention to possible sources of bias, case control studies can provide a valid and efficient method to answer many clinical questions, particularly those involving rare diseases.

Suggested Readings

Cole P: The evolving case-control study. *J Chron Dis*, 1979; 32:15–27.

Feinstein AR: Clinical biostatistics XX: The epidemiologic trohoc, the ablative risk ratio, and 'retrospective research'. *Clin Pharmacol Ther*, 1973; 14:291–307.

Horwitz RI, Feinstein AR: Methodologic standards and contradictory results in case-control research. *Am J Med*, 1979; 66:556–564.

Ibrahim MA, Spitzer WO: The case-control study: The problem and the prospect. *J Chron Dis*, 1979; 32:139–144.

Sartwell PE: Retrospective studies: A review for the clinician. *Ann Int Med*, 1974; 81:381–386.

References

1. National Center for Health Statistics. Prevalence of Selected Chronic Respiratory Conditions: United States 1970. (Series 10, No. 84) U.S. Department of Health, Education, and Welfare, Rockville, Maryland.

2. Lelah T, Harris L, Avery C, Brook R. Asthma in children and adults: Assessing the quality of medical care using short-term outcome measures. In: Quality of Medical Care Assessment Using Outcome Measures: Eight Disease-Specific Applications. Avery A, Lelah T, Solomon N, Harris L, Brook R, Greenfield K, Ware J Jr, Avery C. Santa Monica, CA: Rand Corp, 1976.

3. Fletcher RH, Fletcher SW. Clinical research in general medicine journals: A 30-year perspective. *N Engl J Med*, 1979; 301:180–183.

4. Klatskin G, Kimberg DV. Recurrent hepatitis attributable to halothane sensitization in an anesthetist. *N Engl J Med*, 1969; 280:515–522.

5. Dietz, PE. Sampling bias in the case report: The example of post mortem Cesarean section. Presented at Robert Wood Johnson Clinical Scholars Program National Meeting, 1979.

6. Hetzel P, Gee TS. A new observation in the clinical spectrums of erythroleukemia. *Am J Med*, 1978; 64:765–772.

7. Cole P. The evolving case control study. *J Chron Dis*, 1979; 32:15–27.

8. Boston Collaborative Drug Surveillance Program. Reserpine and breast cancer. *Lancet*, 1974; 2:669–671.

9. Hulka BS, Fowler WC Jr, Kaufman DG, Greenberg BG, Hogue CJR, Berger GS, Pulliam CC. Estrogen and endometrial cancer: Cases and two control groups from North Carolina. *Am J Obstet Gynecol*, 1980; 137:92–101.

10. Sackett DL. Bias in analytic research. *J Chron Dis*, 1979; 32:51–63.

11. Horwitz RI, Feinstein AR. Methodologic standards and contradictory results in case-control research. *Am J Med*, 1979; 66:556–564.

chapter

11

Cause

A few years ago, our medical students were presented a study of the relationship between the cigarette smoking habits of obstetricians and the vigor of babies they delivered. Infant vigor was measured by an Apgar score; a high score (9–10) indicated the baby was healthy while a lower score indicated the baby might be in trouble and require close monitoring. The study suggested that smoking by obstetricians (not in the delivery suite!) had an adverse effect on Apgar scores in newborns (Figure 11.1).

The medical students were then asked to comment on what was wrong with this study, with its unexpected results indicating that obstetricians' smoking caused unhealthy infants. After many suggestions, someone finally said that the conclusion simply did not make sense.

It was then acknowledged that although the study was real, the "exposure" and "disease" had been altered for the presentation. Instead of comparing smoking habits of obstetricians with Apgar scores of newborns, the figure represented a study published in 1843 by Oliver Wendell Holmes (then Professor of Anatomy and Physiology, and later Dean of Harvard Medical School) of hand washing habits by obstetricians and subsequent puerperal sepsis in mothers (Figure 11.2). Although the study by Holmes was not nearly so tidy as Figure 11.2 (the numbers are different and he did not know about cohort and case-control designs nor relative risks and odds ratios), his observations led him to conclude: "The disease known as puerperal fever is so far contagious, as to be frequently carried from patient to patient by physicians and nurses" (1).

One response to Holmes' assertion that unwashed hands caused puerperal fever was remarkably similar to that of the medical student: the findings made no sense. "I prefer to attribute them (puerperal sepsis cases) to accident, or Providence, of which I can form a conception, rather than to contagion of which I cannot form any clear idea, at least as to this particular malady" (1). This response was written by the prestigious

Dr. Charles D. Meigs, Professor of Midwifery and the Diseases of Women and Children at Jefferson Medical College.*

Holmes and Meigs were confronted with the issue of causation. Holmes was convinced by his data that the spread of puerperal sepsis was caused by obstetricians not washing their hands between deliveries. He could not, however, supply the pathogenetic mechanism by which hand washing was related to the disease. Meigs, therefore, remained unconvinced that the cause of puerperal sepsis had been established (and presumably did not bother to wash his hands).

Questions of cause and effect continue to arise, as this modern-day example illustrates.

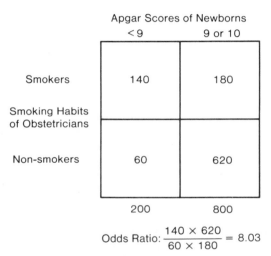

$$\text{Odds Ratio:} \frac{140 \times 620}{60 \times 180} = 8.03$$

Figure 11.1.   Relationship Between Obstetricians' Smoking Habits and Apgar Scores of Newborns.

Example—In the late 1970's, cases of a new and lethal disease, called toxic shock syndrome, began to appear. Patients were usually young women who suffered the onset of fever, rash with desquamation, hypotension, mucous membrane inflammation, and clinical or laboratory evidence of abnormalities affecting many systems. The disease often appeared during menstruation.

Scientists from the Centers for Disease Control began studying the epidemic. In the fall of 1980, representatives of the Food and Drug Administration met with the manufacturer of a new tampon to review data which seemed to show that use of the tampon was associated with many cases of the syndrome. It was not known at the time just how the tampon caused the toxic shock syndrome.

After the review, the manufacturer voluntarily removed the tampon from the market, doing so with little more evidence than Holmes gave Meigs. Upon removal of the tampon from the market, the incidence of the disease declined dramatically (2).

---

* Thanks to Dr. John Hoey, Faculty of Medicine, McGill Medical School for this example.

Clinicians frequently are confronted with information about possible cause-and-effect relationships. In fact, most of this book has been about methods used to establish causation, although we have not called special attention to the term. In this chapter, we will review concepts of cause in clinical medicine. We will then outline the kinds of evidence which, when present, strengthen the likelihood that an association represents a cause-and-effect relationship.

DEFINITION AND CONCEPTS

Webster defines *cause* as "something that brings about an effect or a result" (3). In medical textbooks, cause is usually discussed under such headings as "etiology", "pathogenesis", or "mechanisms."

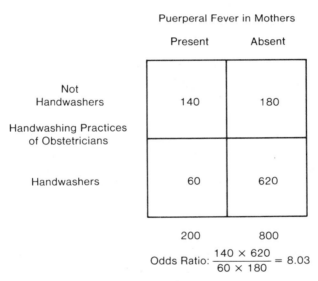

Figure 11.2. Relationship Between Handwashing by Obstetricians and Puerperal Fever in Mothers.

Cause is important to practicing physicians primarily in guiding their approach to three clinical tasks: prevention, diagnosis, and treatment. The clinical examples at the beginning of this chapter illustrate how knowledge of cause-and-effect relationships can lead to successful preventive strategies. Likewise, when we periodically check patients' blood pressures, we are reacting to arguments that hypertension causes morbid and mortal events and that treatment of hypertension causes a reduction in these events. The diagnostic process, especially in infectious disease, frequently involves a search for the causative agent. Less directly, the diagnostic process often depends on information about cause when the presence of risk factors are used to identify groups of patients in whom disease prevalence is high (Chapter 4). Finally, the knowledge of or at least hope for a cause-and-effect relationship underlies every therapeutic maneuver in clinical medicine. Why give penicillin unless we think it will cause a cure of pneumococcal pneumonia? Or why advise a patient with colorectal cancer metastic to the liver to undergo hepatic artery infusion with 5-flurouracil unless we believe the antimetabolite will cause a regression of metastases and a prolongation of survival, comfort, and/or ability to carry on daily activities.

By and large, practitioners are more interested in treatable or reversible than immutable causes. Researchers, on the other hand, might also be interested in studying causal factors for which no efficacious treatment or prevention exists in hopes of developing future preventions and treatments.

Single and Multiple Causes

In 1882, 40 years after the Holmes-Meigs confrontation, Koch set forth his postulates for determining that an infectious agent is the cause of a disease:

1. The organism must be present in every case of the disease.
2. The organism must be isolated and grown in pure culture.
3. The organism must, when innoculated into a susceptible animal, cause the specific disease.
4. The organism must then be recovered from the animal and identified.

Koch's postulates contributed greatly to the concept of cause in medicine. Before Koch, it was believed that many different bacteria caused any given disease. The application of his postulates helped bring order out of chaos, and allowed for important scientific advances. They are still useful today. For example, Koch's postulates were the basis for the statement in 1977 that Legionnaire's disease is caused by a gram negative bacterium.

The causes of many diseases, however, cannot be established by means of Koch's postulates. Basic to his approach was that a particular disease had one cause, and a particular cause results in one disease. Would that all diseases were so simple! Smoking causes lung cancer, chronic obstructive pulmonary disease, peptic ulcers, bladder cancer, and coronary artery disease. On the other hand, coronary artery disease has multiple causes, including cigarette smoking, hypertension, and hypercholesterolemia. It is also possible to have coronary artery disease without any of these known risk factors being present.

Thus, for most diseases, there are many causes; and a causal factor for any one disease often results in many other diseases as well. In fact, usually many factors act together to cause disease. This process has been called the "web of causation" (4). Koch's postulates are useful only in those special circumstances in which one particular cause dominates (perhaps because the other determinants of disease are already present, but insufficient in themselves to cause disease) and when that cause is physically transmissible.

Interaction of Multiple Causes

When more than one cause act together, their effects are not necessarily simply additive. Often, the resulting risk is greater than would be expected by simply adding the effects of the separate causes.

Example—Figure 11.3 shows that probability of developing cardiovascular disease over an eight-year period among men aged 40. Those men who did not smoke cigarettes, had low serum cholesterol values, and had low systolic blood pressure readings were at low risk of developing disease (12/1000). Risk increased,

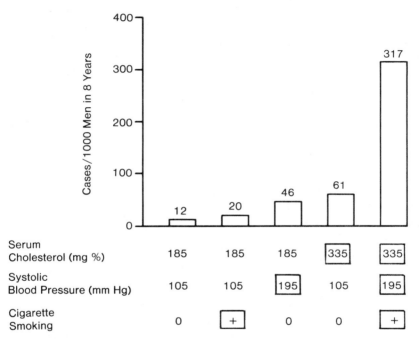

Figure 11.3. Interaction of Separate Causes of Disease: Risk of Developing Cardiovascular Disease in Men, According to Levels of Several Risk Factors, Alone and in Combination. Abnormal values are enclosed in boxes. (Drawn from: Kannel WB. *Postgrad Med*, 1977; 61:74–85.)

in the range of 20 to 61/1000, when the various factors were present individually. But when all three factors were present, the risk of cardiovascular disease (317/1000) was almost three times greater than the sum of the individual risks (5).

Elucidation of cause is more difficult when many factors play a part than when a single one predominates. However, when multiple causative factors are present, and interact, it may be possible to make a substantial impact on a patient's health by changing only one, or a small number, of the causes. Thus, in the previous example, getting patients to give up smoking and treating hypertension might substantially lower the risk of developing cardiovascular disease in men, even in the continuing presence of other causative factors. (Studies are underway to determine if this is indeed so.)

Proximity of Cause to Effect

When biomedical scientists study causes of disease, they usually search for the underlying pathogenetic mechanism or final common pathway of disease. It is our impression that most clinicians accept this as the fundamental approach to determining cause-and-effect relationships. Certainly basic biomedical research aimed at elucidating pathogenetic causes of disease has played a crucial part in the advancement of medical science in this century. However, the occurrence of disease is also determined by less specific, more remote causes such as genetic, environmental, or behavioral factors, which occur earlier in the chain of events

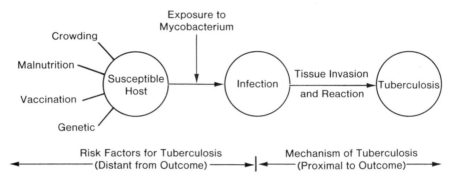

Figure 11.4.   Causes of Tuberculosis.

leading to a disease. These are sometimes referred to as "origins" of disease and are more likely to be investigated by epidemiologists. These less specific and more remote causes of disease are the risk factors discussed in Chapter 6.

It is important to understand the contribution of these two ways of considering cause. Unfortunately, if the pathogenetic mechanism is not clear, it is sometimes assumed that the cause of a disease is not known. But, in such situations, knowledge of risk factors may lead to very effective treatments and preventions which can be applied without knowing the pathogenetic mechanism of a disease. (Thus, Holmes was right in his assertion that obstetricians should wash their hands, even though he had little notion of bacteria.) To view cause in medicine exclusively as cellular and subcellular processes restricts the possibilities for useful clinical interventions.

The following is an example of a disease with a rich array of causes, most of which are amenable to interventions that either prevent or reverse the disease.

Example—Koch's postulates were originally used to establish that tuberculosis is caused by innoculation of the acid fast bacillus, mycobacterium tuberculosis, into susceptible hosts. The final common pathway of tuberculosis is the invasion of host tissue by the bacteria. From a pathogenetic perspective, conquering the disease required antibiotics or vaccines which were effective against the organism. Through biomedical research efforts, both have been developed.

However, the development of the disease, tuberculosis, is far more complex. Other important causes are the degree of susceptibility of the host and the degree of exposure (Figure 11.4). In fact, these causes determine whether invasion of host tissue can occur.

Some clinicians would be hesitant to label host susceptibility and level of exposure as causes of tuberculosis, but they are very important components of cause. In fact, social and economic factors influencing host susceptibility may have played a more prominent role in controlling tuberculosis than treatments

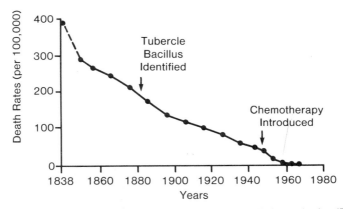

Figure 11.5. Declining Death Rate from Respiratory Tuberculosis. (Redrawn from: McKeown T. The Role of Medicine: Dream, Mirage, or Nemesis. London: Nuffield Provincial Hospitals Trust, 1976.)

developed through the biomedical-pathogenetic research model. Figure 11.5 shows that the death rate from tuberculosis had dropped dramatically long before antibiotics were introduced. (Vaccine came even later.)

Another example of the importance of both pathogenetic and epidemiologic approaches to cause is the recent decline in deaths from coronary artery disease in the United States. Over the past decade, the death rate from coronary artery disease has dropped approximately 25%. This decline accompanied decreased exposure, in the population as a whole, to several apparent causes of cardiovascular disease. A larger proportion of people with hypertension are being treated effectively, middle-aged men are smoking less, and cholesterol consumption has declined. These developments were, at least in part, the result of both epidemiologic and biomedical studies, and have spared tens of thousands of lives per year. It is doubtful they would have occurred without the understanding of both the proximal mechanisms and the more remote origins of cardiovascular disease.

ESTABLISHING CAUSE

In clinical medicine, it is not possible to prove causal relationships beyond any doubt. It is only possible to increase one's conviction of a cause-and-effect relationship, by means of empirical evidence, to the point where, for all intents and purposes, cause is established. Conversely, evidence against a cause can be mounted until a cause-and-effect relationship becomes implausible.

These principles are true even for clinical applications of well-established laboratory findings. Although more certainty can be attached to observations made in the laboratory under highly controlled conditions, a biologic mechanism established in the laboratory cannot be assumed to apply in intact patients. The particular mechanism which is characterized under carefully controlled conditions may be overpowered by other, competing mechanisms which are not yet understood.

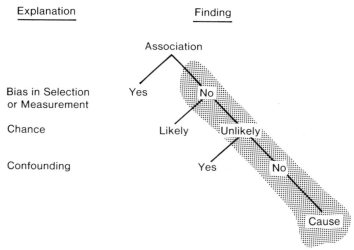

Figure 11.6.   Explanation of an Association: Bias, Chance, Confounding and Cause.

The following is an example of a causal hypothesis, suggested in the laboratory and not supported by clinical research.

Example—Platelet aggregation, which takes place during thrombotic events, can be prevented by aspirin. Because platelet aggregation is involved in the development of myocardial infarctions, it was thought that reinfarctions might be prevented by giving aspirin to patients who had experienced recent myocardial infarctions. However, a randomized controlled trial of aspirin demonstrated no protective effect. It is likely that the effect of aspirin on platelets, demonstrated in laboratory tests, was overshadowed by other factors contributing to the development of reinfarctions (6).

Cause-and-effect relationships for humans, therefore, must ultimately be established in intact humans. In order to do so, the possibility of a postulated cause-and-effect relationship should be examined in as many different ways as possible.

Association and Cause

Two factors obviously must appear to be associated if they are to be considered cause-and-effect. However, not all associations are causal. Figure 11.6 outlines other kinds of associations that must be excluded. First, a decision must be made as to whether an apparent association between a purported cause and an effect is real, or merely an artifact because of bias or random variation. Selection and measurement biases and the role of chance are most likely to give rise to apparent associations, which in reality do not exist. If these problems can be considered unlikely, an association exists. But before deciding that the association is causal,

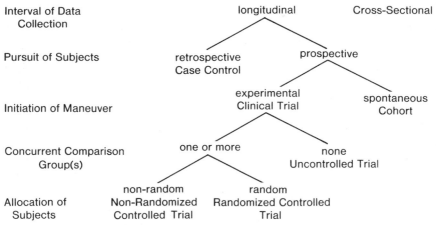

Figure 11.7. Summary of Research Designs Used to Establish Cause.

it is necessary to know if the association occurs indirectly, through another (confounding) factor, or directly. If confounding is not found, a causal relationship is likely. However, one should always keep in mind that at some future time another factor may be found which is more directly causal. For example, when it was found that jaundice followed injection of neoarsphenamine for syphilis, the drug was considered responsible. Later, the jaundice was found to be secondary to hepatitis resulting from the use of unclean syringes to inject neoarsphenamine, not the drug itself. Thus, factors which are considered causes at one time are sometimes found to be indirectly related to disease later, when more evidence is available.

Design of the Clinical Investigation

The most important evidence for establishing a cause-and-effect relationship is the strength of the research design used to establish the relationship. Figure 11.7 is a summary of research designs used in clinical investigation and described in preceding chapters. (Case reports, which are not included, can be conducted using any of the designs, but their usefulness in establishing cause is limited because they report the experience of only a small number of patients, so that the results could easily represent bias or chance.)

Well-conducted randomized controlled trials, with adequate numbers of patients, blinding of therapists, patients, and researchers, and carefully standardized methods of measurement and analysis, are the best evidence for a cause-and-effect relationship. As pointed out in Chapter 8, the reason why randomized controlled trials are the most powerful way of establishing cause-and-effect relationships in clinical investigations is that they are best suited to study the unique effects of a single factor. They guard against differences in the groups being compared, both for factors already known to be important, which can be overcome by means other than a randomized controlled trial, and for unknown confounding factors which have not yet been identified.

We ordinarily use randomized controlled trials to provide evidence about cause-and-effect relationships for treatments and preventions. At least theoretically, such trials could also be used to show a particular agent causes a disease. However, it is usually not possible to use them for this purpose. While potentially helpful agents may be assigned at random, at least to some patients, most potentially harmful agents or risk factors cannot. Such studies would be unethical, because patients who enter them could only do worse than they would have done without the trial. Moreover, even the removal of potential risk factors is rarely possible. For example, although one can randomize laboratory animals to smoking and non-smoking groups, it is certainly not possible to do so with humans. Then too, there are problems of long latent periods and large numbers of subjects needed to answer most questions about cause-and-effect relationships in clinical medicine.

Because of all these problems, randomized controlled trials are rarely feasible when studying causes of disease. Observational studies must be used.

In general, the further down Figure 11.7, the better the research design protects against possible biases, and the stronger the evidence is for a cause-and-effect relationship. Well-conducted cohort studies are the next best thing to experiments, because they can be conducted to minimize the effects of selection and measurement biases, as well as known confounding biases. Cross-sectional studies are vulnerable because they provide no direct evidence of the sequence of events. True prevalence surveys, cross-sectional studies of a defined population, guard against selection bias, but are subject to measurement and confounding biases. As pointed out in Chapter 10, case control studies are vulnerable to selection bias as well. Weakest of all are cases series which are cross-sectional studies with no defined population and no comparison group.

Of course, the hierarchy depicted in Figure 11.7 is only a rough guide, based on extent of susceptibility to bias. The manner in which an individual study is performed can do a great deal to increase or decrease its validity, regardless of the type of design used.

Temporal Relationships between Cause and Effect

Causes should obviously precede effects. When this is clearly not so, a cause-and-effect relationship is not possible.

This fundamental principle seems self-evident, but it can be overlooked when interpreting cross-sectional studies and some case control studies, in which both purported causes and effects are measured at the same point in time. In these two types of studies, it is often assumed that one variable precedes another without actually establishing that this is so. The controversy about whether estrogen therapy causes endometrial cancer is an example of this problem, as pointed out in Chapter 10. Some investigators argue that the assumption in case control studies that estrogen therapy leads to endometrial cancer, which then becomes manifest by postmenopausal uterine bleeding, may be in error. They argue that because exogenous estrogens are used to treat postmenopausal bleeding, it is possible that endometrial cancer causes uterine bleeding which then leads to estrogen therapy being prescribed. If the endometrial cancer is diagnosed after estrogen therapy is begun, it would then seem that estrogens preceded the cancer, but such a conclusion would be incorrect. (Subsequent studies have shown that the latter possibility could not explain all of the observed odds ratio, but the example does illustrate that temporal sequence may not be clear in non-cohort studies of cause-and-effect relationships.)

Although it is absolutely necessary for a cause to precede an effect, it is important to keep in mind that temporal sequence alone is weak evidence for cause. In particular, measuring an effect only once before and only once after exposure to a suspected cause is open to many interpretations.

Evidence that a factor is actually responsible for an effect can be strengthened if observations are made at more than two points in time (before and after) and in more than one place. In a *time series study*, the effect is measured at various points in time before and after the purported cause has been introduced. It is then possible to see if the effect varies in a similar fashion. If changes in the purported cause are followed by changes in the purported effect, the association is less likely to be spurious, especially if the association between cause and effect is maintained both while the cause is increasing and decreasing.

Example—The frequency of toxic shock syndrome, discussed at the beginning of this chapter, is illustrated in Figure 11.8. The tampon suspected of causing toxic shock syndrome was introduced to the market in August 1978 and removed from the market in September 1980. The frequency of reported cases of toxic shock syndrome in the United States varied according to the introduction and withdrawal of the product (2).

In a *multiple time-series study*, the purported cause has been introduced into several different groups at various times. Measurements of effect are then made among the groups to determine if the effect occurs in the same sequential manner in which the purported cause was introduced.

Example—Because there have been no randomized controlled trials of cervical cancer screening programs, their effectiveness has been evaluated by means of a multiple time series. Data were gathered on the screening programs begun in the various Canadian provinces. As can be seen in Table 11.1, the extent of screening varied from province to province over a 10-year period. Screening was well underway in British Columbia in 1962; by 1967, it was underway in Alberta, Saskatchewan, Manitoba, Ontario, and Nova Scotia. By 1971, programs were active in Quebec, New Brunswick, Prince Edward Island, and Newfoundland.

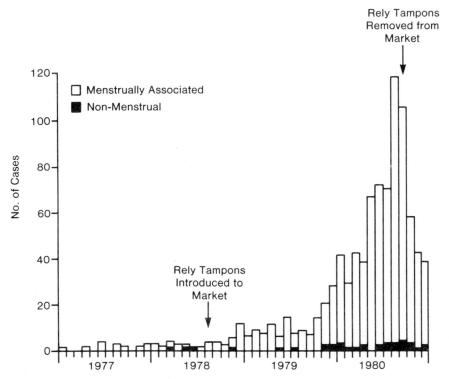

Figure 11.8.   Example of a Time Series Study: Reported Cases of Toxic-Shock Syndrome in the United States, January 1977 through December 1980, in Relation to the Marketing of Rely Tampons. (Redrawn from: *Morbid Mortal Rep*, 1981; 30:25–28.)

Figure 11.9 shows the changes in mortality from carcinoma of the cervix in these same provinces over the period of time during which screening programs became active. Changes in mortality followed the introduction of screening programs, regardless of time or location. With these data, it was concluded that "screening has had a significant effect on reduction in mortality from carcinoma of the uterus" (7).

Studies like the ones just cited are called *ecological studies*; exposure and disease were both measured in populations rather than in individuals. It is possible, therefore, that the individuals who were exposed were not the ones who got the disease. For this reason, a times series study alone cannot be regarded as strong evidence for cause-and-effect. Multiple time series studies are stronger evidence for causal relationships because it is unlikely that bias would act in the same direction, to the same extent, in several times and places.

Strength of the Association

A strong association between a purported cause and an effect, as expressed by a large relative risk or odds ratio, is better evidence for a

Table 11.1

Extent of Cervical Cancer Screening in the Canadian Provinces in 1962, 1967, and 1971*

Province	No. of Cytologic Examinations as % of Female Population Aged 20 Years or More		
	1962	1967	1971
British Columbia	23	41	55
Alberta	5	27	40
Saskatchewan	1	24	41
Manitoba	7	22	46
Ontario	3	22	39
Quebec	3	13	29
New Brunswick	2	13	22
Nova Scotia	7	24	37
Prince Edward Island	1	13	28
Newfoundland	1	14	36

* Data from Cervical Cancer Screening Programs. *Canad Med Assoc J* 1976; 114:1003–1030.

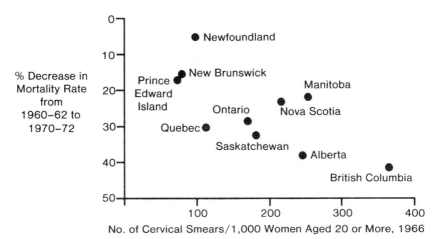

Figure 11.9. Example of a Multiple Time Series Study: The Change in Mortality from Carcinoma of the Cervix in Relation to Screening Rates in Canadian Provinces. (Redrawn from: Cervical Cancer Screening Programs. *Canad Med Assoc J*, 1976; 114:1003–1030.)

causal relationship than a weak association. Thus, the four- to 16-fold increase of lung cancer among smokers, compared to non-smokers, in eight different prospective studies is much stronger evidence that smoking causes lung cancer than the findings in these same studies that smoking may be related to renal cancer, where the relative risks are much smaller (1.1–1.6) (8). Bias can result in even very large relative risks. However, unrecognized bias is less likely to produce large relative risks than small ones.

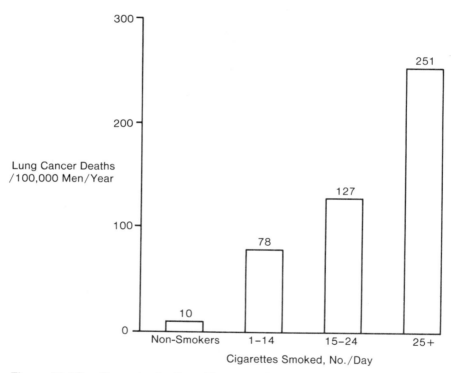

Figure 11.10.   Example of a Dose-Response Relationship Between Cause and Effect: Lung Cancer Death "Responses" According to Cigarette "Doses" in Male Physicians. (Drawn from: Doll R, Peto R. *Br Med J*, 1976; 2:1525–1536.)

Dose-Response Relationships

A dose-response relationship is present when varying amounts of the purported cause are related to varying amounts of the effect. If a dose-response relationship can be demonstrated, it strengthens the argument for cause and effect. Figure 11.10 shows a clear dose-response curve when lung cancer death rates (responses) are plotted against number of cigarettes smoked (doses).

Although a dose-response curve is good evidence for a causal relationship, especially when coupled with a large relative risk, the relationship can be the result of bias. Whether this is likely or not depends on the clinical characteristics of the disease in question, as the following example illustrates.

Example—The estrogen/endometrial cancer and cigarette smoking/lung cancer associations illustrate the importance of knowing the clinical characteristics of diseases when evaluating the possibility of a selection bias. For both of these associations, a dose-response curve has been documented. [For estrogen and endometrial cancer, a relationship exists between the duration of exogenous estrogen use and the risk of developing endometrial cancer (9)]. It has been argued that this association appears because estrogen simply unmasks endometrial cancer by provoking increased bleeding (10). According to this argument, endometrial cancer is equally present among women who do not take estrogen, but in them the cancer remains asymptomatic and unsuspected. Such an argument hinges on the assertion that endometrial cancer can remain asymptomatic for extended periods of time, and it is at least clinically plausible for this kind of slow growing cancer.

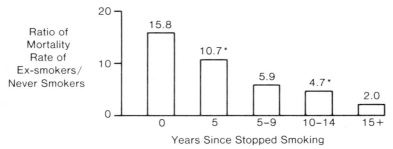

Figure 11.11. A Reversible Association: Decreasing Mortality from Lung Cancer in Ex-Cigarette Smokers Among British Doctors. * Excludes people who stopped smoking after getting cancer. (Drawn from: Doll R, Peto R. *Br Med J*, 1976; 2:1525–1536.)

On the other hand, the same kind of bias is not a clinically plausible explanation for the association between smoking and lung cancer. It is not reasonable to assume that lung cancer remains asymptomatic among non-smokers; clinical experience suggests that this disease is rapidly fatal, with a very short asymptomatic period.

The existence of a dose-response relationship between exposure and disease also does not exclude confounding. For instance, both the strong association between smoking and lung cancer and the dose-response relationship have been dismissed by the tobacco industry as examples of confounding. According to this argument, there is some unknown variable (X) which both causes people to smoke and increases their risk of developing lung cancer. The more the factor is present, the more both smoking and lung cancer are found—hence, the dose-response relationship. Such an argument is a theoretically plausible explanation for the association between smoking and lung cancer. Short of a randomized controlled trial (which would, on the average, allocate the people with confounding variable equally to smoking and non-smoking groups), it is a difficult argument to refute.

Reversible Associations

A factor is more likely to be a cause of disease if its removal results in a decreased risk of disease—i.e., the association between purported cause and effect is reversible. For example, people who give up smoking decrease their likelihood of getting lung cancer (Figure 11.11). Nevertheless, confounding can still explain a reversible association. For example, it is still possible that people willing to give up smoking have smaller amounts of the X variable than those who continue to smoke.

Consistency

When several studies, conducted at different times in different settings and with different patients, all come to the same conclusion, evidence for a causal relationship is strengthened. However, several studies may all make the same mistake. So causation is particularly supported when studies conducted using several different research designs all lead to the same result.

It is often the case that different studies produce different results. Lack of consistency does not necessarily mean the results of a particular study are invalid. One good study should outweigh several poor ones. Thus, as pointed out in Chapter 1, well-conducted studies supporting the efficacy of Bacille Calmette-Guerin (BCG) vaccinations in preventing tuberculosis deserve more weight than the less well-conducted studies showing no protective effect.

Biologic Plausibility

The biologic plausibility of a purported cause-and-effect association (Meig's and the medical student's criterion) is often given considerable weight when assessing causation. Biologic plausibility rests on whether the assertion of cause-and-effect is consistent with our knowledge of the mechanisms of disease as they are currently understood. When we have absolutely no idea how an association might have arisen, we tend to be skeptical that the association is real. Such skepticism often serves us well. For example, the substance, Laetrile, has been touted as a cure for cancer. However, the scientific community was not convinced that Laetrile would have a beneficial effect on cancer patients. They could think of no biologic reason why it should because the substance is an extract of apricot pits and not chemically related to compounds with known anticancer activity. To "nail down" the issue, Laetrile was finally submitted to a randomized controlled trial in which it was shown that the substance was, in fact, without activity against the cancers studied (11).

It is important to remember, however, that what is considered biologically plausible depends on the state of medical knowledge at the time. In Meig's day, contagious diseases were biologically implausible. Today, a biologically plausible mechanism for toxic shock syndrome, the action of an exotoxin produced by Staphylococcus aureus has been proposed, and this has made it easier for us to accept the epidemiologic data. On the other hand, the mechanism by which acupuncture causes anesthesia is far less clear. To many, the suggestion that anesthesia is caused by sticking needles into the body and twirling them seems biologically implausible, and so they do not believe in the effectiveness of acupuncture.

In sum, biologic plausibility, when present, strengthens the case for causation. When it is absent, other evidence for causation should be sought. If the other evidence is strong, the lack of biologic plausibility may indicate the limitations of medical knowledge rather than the lack of a causal association.

Table 11.2
Grading Types of Clinical Evidence for a Cause-and-Effect Relationship

Grade	Type of Evidence
Strong	Randomized controlled trial
	Cohort study
	Multiple time series
Medium	Large relative risk or odds ratio
	Dose-response relationship
	Reversible association
	Case control study
	Time-series
Weak	Correct temporal sequence
	Cross-sectional study
	Small relative risk or odds ratio
	Biologic plausibility
	Consistency of results

"Grading" the Evidence

A cause-and-effect relationship is more likely when many lines of evidence all lead to the same conclusion. If an association is biologically plausible, has a large relative risk, demonstrates a dose-response relationship and a reversible relationship, and has been found to be present in many different sites and by means of various study designs, the case for a causal association is much stronger than if the results of some of the studies are contrary to the causal hypothesis.

When evidence is conflicting, as is often the case, the clinician must decide where the weight of the evidence lies. Table 11.2 summarizes the different types of evidence for cause, and indicates the relative strength of a positive result in helping to establish or discard a causal hypothesis.

SUMMARY

Cause-and-effect relationships underlie diagnostic, preventive, and therapeutic activities in clinical medicine.

Diseases usually have many causes, although occasionally one might predominate. Often several causes interact with one another in such a way that the risk of disease is more than would be expected by simply adding up the effects of the individual causes taken separately.

Causes of disease can be proximal pathogenetic mechanisms or more remote genetic, environmental, or behavioral factors. Medical interventions to prevent or reverse disease can occur at any place in the development of disease, from remote origins to proximal mechanisms.

The case for causation rests primarily on the strength of the research designs used to establish it. Because we rarely have the opportunity to establish cause using randomized controlled trials, observational studies are necessary. In such cases, factors which strengthen the argument for a cause-and-effect relationship include temporal relationships, the strength of the association between cause and effect, the existence of a dose-response relationship, a fall in risk when the purported cause is removed, and consistency of results from several studies. Biologic plausibility, and coherence with known facts are other features that help to establish cause.

Suggested Readings

Hill AB. Chapter 24. Statistical evidence and inference. In: Principles of Medical Statistics. New York: Oxford University Press, 1966.

Murphy EA. Cause: A theoretical approach; Cause: A practical approach. In: The Logic of Medicine. Chapters 7 and 14. Baltimore: The Johns Hopkins University Press, 1976.

MacMahon B, Pugh TF. Chapter 2. Concepts of Cause. In: Epidemiology: Principles and Methods. Boston: Little, Brown and Company, 1970.

Buck C. Popper's philosophy for epidemiologists. *Int J Epid*, 1975; 4:159.

Rothman KJ. Reviews and commentary. Causes. *Am J Epid*, 1976; 104:587–592.

References

1. Holmes OW. On the contagiousness of puerperal fever. New Engl Quart J of Med and Surg 1843. *In:* Medical Classics 1936; 1:207–268.
2. Morbidity and Mortality Weekly Report. 1981; 30:25–28.
3. Webster's New Collegiate Dictionary. Springfield: C.G. Merriam Company, 1977.
4. MacMahon B, Pugh TF. Epidemiology. Principles and Methods. Boston: Little, Brown, and Company, 1970.
5. Kannel WB. Preventive cardiology. *Postgrad Med*, 1977; 61:74–85.
6. Aspirin Myocardial Infarction Study Research Group: A randomized controlled trial of aspirin in persons recovered from myocardial infarction. *JAMA*, 1980; 243:661–669.
7. Cervical Cancer Screening Programs. *Can Med Assoc J*, 1976; 114:1003–1033.
8. Morbidity and Mortality Weekly Report. 1979; 28:1–11.
9. Hulka BS, Grimson RG, Greenberg BG, Kaufman DG, Fowler WC Jr, Hogue CJR, Berger GS, Pulliam CC. "Alternative" controls in a case-control study of endometrial cancer and exogenous estrogen. *Am J Epid*, 1980; 112:376–378.
10. Horwitz RI, Feinstein AR. Alternative analytic methods for case-control studies of estrogens and endometrial cancer. *N Engl J Med*, 1978; 299:1089–1094.
11. Moertel, CG, Fleming TR, Rubin J, Kvols LK, Sarna G, Koch R, Currie VE, Young CW, Jones SE, Davignon JP. A clinical trial of amygdalin (laetrile) in the treatment of human cancer. *N Engl J Med*, 1982; 301:201–206.

chapter

12

Summing Up

A major theme of this book is that collective clinical experience, whether reported in hospital corridors or published in the medical literature, must be viewed critically and cautiously before it is used to alter clinical practice. Two questions frequently are raised in response to this plea for critical caution:

Can I not trust the authors and editors of medical textbooks and journals?

Can I really be expected to decide on my own which data or conclusions are valid?

Put simply, our response is NO to the first question and YES to the second.

We are not suggesting that medical authors and editors are dishonest, dumb, deceitful, or anything of the sort. The historical fact, however, is that biased results abound in the medical literature, as evidenced by the plethora of useless diagnostic maneuvers and therapies which are continually being introduced and then purged from medical practice. In part, this reflects the recency of a more widespread appreciation of epidemiologic research designs and other methods in clinical research. For example, although randomized controlled clinical trials seem so intuitively logical, they were not used to examine medical therapy until the 1950's. It also reflects the often overlooked fact that authors and editors are human, excited by new and positive findings, not wanting to be left out of important developments, enthusiastic about what they are doing to help stamp out pain and suffering. Whatever the reason, clinical readers must exercise independent critical judgment in deciding which research findings will influence the care of their patients. At the very least, the clinician must resolve those medical controversies which touch day-to-day practice.

This chapter illustrates the application of principles outlined in earlier chapters. We have chosen as an example one of the most heated and long-lasting controversies in Internal Medicine, the debate over the cardiotoxicity of oral hypoglycemic agents. Our purpose is not to conclude that debate, but to show how the principles of clinical epidemiology can be used by informed clinicians to assess the studies on their own.

Let us begin with a patient who poses the problem.

Ms. HC is a 56-year-old woman who has come to her physician because of polydipsia and polyuria. Physical examination reveals obesity and no complications of diabetes. Urine glucose is 3+ by glucose oxidase test and a two-hour postprandial blood glucose is 280 mg/dl. Urine ketones are persistently negative.

She is placed on a weight reduction diet and followed closely. After an initial 10-lb weight loss, her weight remains steady and her urine glucoses continue to be elevated. She expresses considerable anxiety about giving herself injections and asks whether she could have pills instead.

The problem represented by this patient is whether oral hypoglycemic agents present a reasonable alternative to insulin. A logical first place to pursue this issue is to examine current textbooks.

"Although weight reduction by caloric restriction is the ideal approach to the middle-aged overweight diabetic subject, it is almost universally unsuccessful. Thus, in these patients, as well as in non-overweight subjects with maturity-onset type diabetes, addition of the oral hypoglycemic agents is indicated should hyperglycemia persist, although, as discussed below, some controversy exists among experts in the field as to their value and contraindications.

In a large multicenter study, the University Group Diabetes Project, sponsored by the National Institutes of Health and performed through the 1960's, it was demonstrated that middle-aged subjects on a fixed dose of the sulfonylurea, Tolbutamide, although showing a small but significant lowering of blood glucose levels, had an increased incidence of sudden death, presumably resulting from myocardial infarction or arrhythmia. This study has limited the indiscriminate use of sulfonylureas, and has placed further emphasis on diet as the primary approach to the maturity-onset type of diabetic. Many experienced students of the disease question the significance of the study and continue to use the agents. Nevertheless, if one adheres to the hypothesis that hyperglycemia is deleterious, in that it leads to the microvascular complications, then the sulfonylureas may be indicated if their benefit outweighs the possible risk of increased myocardial instability. Certainly, in the elderly female with glycosuria, the correction of her discomfort associated with the glycosuria may far outweigh the theoretical increased risk of sudden death as found in the UGDP study."

Cecil's Textbook of Medicine, 1979

"Maturity-onset diabetes that cannot be controlled by careful dietary management usually responds to sulfonylureas. The drugs are convenient to use and work in a high percentage of cases. However, some physicians no longer use them because the University Group Diabetes Program (UGDP) cooperative study concluded that Tolbutamide was no more effective than diet alone in the treatment of diabetes and that patients treated with Tolbutamide had a significant increase in cardiac deaths when compared with controls. The validity of the UGDP study has been widely debated, but the evidence pro and con is too extensive to be reviewed here. Suffice it to say that many physicians continue to believe that the sulfonylureas are useful and safe drugs for the treatment of certain adult-onset diabetes."

Harrison's Principles of Internal Medicine, 1980

Both textbooks indicate that controversy persists and that it stems from the varying views as to the "significance" or "validity" of the UGDP study. Is the increased incidence of "sudden" or "cardiac" deaths real or merely "possible", "theoretical", or simply fallacious? Moreover, these passages also state that "many experienced students of the disease question the significance of the study" or "many physicians continue to believe that the sulfonylureas are useful and safe," suggesting that the UGDP findings are open to serious question.

Because the textbooks do not clearly recommend for or against the use of oral agents and the decision seems to hinge on the interpretation of one study, concerned physicians have no recourse but to examine the UGDP findings and related papers for themselves.

WHAT WAS THE UGDP STUDY?

The UGDP (University Group Diabetes Program) study set out to answer the question of whether better control of elevated blood sugar could reduce or retard the incidence of vascular complications in maturity-onset, non-ketosis prone diabetics (1). To answer the question, they organized a multicenter randomized controlled clinical trial illustrated in Figure 12.1.

Twelve clinics initially participated. They recruited recently diagnosed (within one year) adult diabetic patients who did not show evidence of ketosis and whose physicians believed that they had a life expectancy of at least five years. After a one-month period of dietary therapy alone, patients not exhibiting ketosis or other serious complications were randomized, separately in each of the 12 clinics, into four treatment groups. The Tolbutamide (TOLB) group received a fixed dose of Tolbutamide, 500 mg three times a day, whereas the placebo group (PLBO) received an inert tablet of similar appearance three times daily. A third group (ISTD) received a standard, fixed dose of insulin daily, whereas the fourth group (IVAR) received variable amounts of insulin adjusted to maintain good blood sugar control. Patients were then assessed every three months for the occurrence of vascular complications.

After eight years, the mortality experience of the four treatment groups indicated an excess of deaths in the TOLB group as compared with the PLBO group, as shown in Table 12.1. The excess in all deaths did not reach statistical significance ($p = 0.17$), but the excess in deaths from cardiovascular (CVD) causes was highly statistically significant ($p = 0.005$). Because of concerns for the safety of its subjects, the UGDP decided to discontinue the use of TOLB and report these preliminary findings.

CRITICISMS OF THE UGDP STUDY

The presentation of the previous results and the Group's conclusion that TOLB was probably responsible for the excess deaths began a vociferous, even acrimonious, debate which continues to the present. UGDP's critics have mustered a variety of arguments, the most relevant of which proffer reasons why the findings are invalid (2–6). Table 12.2 summarizes seven frequently encountered criticisms of the study that

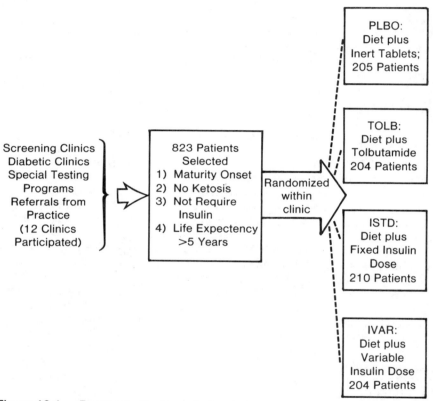

Figure 12.1. Research Design of the UGDP Randomized Clinical Trial. (Adapted from University Group Diabetes Program. *Diabetes.* 1970; 19 (Suppl 2):747–783.)

could threaten the validity of its findings. To understand the importance of these criticisms, each should be recast so as to question the influence of the putative flaw on the findings of excess deaths in the TOLB group. For example, the fact (and it is a fact) that some individuals were entered into the trial even though they did not meet the study's defined criteria for diabetes has particular relevance if their inclusion somehow increased the death rate in the TOLB group or decreased the death rates in the other groups. The same must be asked of all the criticisms.

The seven criticisms outlined in Table 12.2 suggest biases of the sort discussed throughout this book. For example, selection bias becomes a possibility by the inclusion of non-diabetics, the involvement of clinics with particularly sick patients, or the selection of a "peculiarly" healthy PLBO group. Measurement bias is suggested by the criticism that the experience of treatment dropouts was counted in their original group even though they may have received the assigned treatment for only a

Table 12.1

Number and Percentage of Deaths in Each Treatment Group by Cause of Death*

	PLBO	TOLB	ISTD	IVAR
Number at risk of death	205	204	210	204
Number of deaths from cardiovascular causes				
1. Myocardial infarction	0	10	3	2
2. Sudden death	4	4	4	5
3. Other heart disease	1	5	1	2
4. Extracardiac vascular disease	5	7	5	3
All CV causes	10	26	13	12
Number of deaths from non-cardiovascular causes				
5. Cancer	7	2	4	2
6. Cause other than 1–5	3	2	2	3
7. Unknown Cause	1	0	1	1
Number of deaths from all causes	21	30	20	18
Percentage dead from:				
CVD Causes (%)	4.9	12.7	6.2	5.9
All Causes (%)	10.2	14.7	9.5	8.8

* Adapted from University Group Diabetes Program, *Diabetes* 1970; 19 (suppl 2):785–830.

short time. The allegation that the TOLB group was at higher risk of cardiovascular disease suggests that the effect of TOLB on mortality was confounded by the effect of known cardiovascular risk factors.

For the physician caring for Ms. HC, the question is whether an enlightened reader can decide if these potential problems have, in fact, biased the findings and unfairly maligned TOLB treatment. Fortunately, between publications of the UGDP (1, 7) and re-analyses of their results by other interested parties (8, 9), the published literature provides some help in resolving the questions. From these sources, data are available bearing on each of the criticisms. Complex mathematics were rarely necessary, as indicated in the subsequent tables which depend almost exclusively on the stratification of the groups into relevant subgroups. This simple technique, described in Chapter 7, permits straightforward visual evaluation of the effect of a characteristic on the findings.

Table 12.2
Criticisms of the UGDP Study

1. Patients were entered who did not meet the criteria for diabetes.
2. The use of a fixed dose of tolbutamide (or insulin) is inconsistent with clinical practice.
3. The deaths of patients who stopped or switched their treatment were counted in their original group.
4. Why wasn't there a statistically significant increased risk of total mortality in the TOLB group?
5. The 12 clinics were very different with most of the deaths occurring in a few clinics.
6. The randomization was bad and more high risk subjects ended up in the TOLB group. In addition, they did not measure smoking histories.
7. The PLBO group had a 'spuriously' low cardiovascular mortality.

Table 12.3
Number and Percentage of Deaths in Each Treatment Group Before and After Exclusion of Patients Not Meeting Study Entry Criteria*

	PLBO	TOLB	ISTD	IVAR
Number randomized	205	204	210	204
Deaths	21	30	20	18
Percentage Dead (%)	10.2	14.7	9.5	8.8
Patients not meeting criteria	10	19	17	13
Deaths	1	0	0	0
Patients meeting criteria	195	185	193	191
Deaths	20	30	20	18
Percentage dead (%)	10.3	16.2	10.4	9.4

* Adapted from University Group Diabetes Program. *Diabetes* 1970; 19 (Suppl 2):747–783.

Criticism 1—The Inclusion of Patients Not Meeting the Study Criteria

The inclusion of 59 patients who failed to meet the defined criteria for diabetes is sloppy research execution, but does it invalidate the findings? That would depend on whether these potentially low risk patients were disproportionately allocated to the PLBO group. Table 12.3 demonstrates the group allocation and mortality experience of these 59 patients. In fact, nearly twice as many "non-diabetics" were randomized to the TOLB group, as compared to the PLBO group and, as expected, their mortality was low. The *lower section* of Table 12.3 shows that the exclusion of these inappropriately entered patients actually increases the total mortality rate in the TOLB group while slightly lowering it in the PLBO group, reducing the p value of the difference nearly to p = 0.05. Thus, the inclusion of inappropriate subjects can in no way account for the differences in mortality. If anything, their inclusion in the study tended to reduce the mortality excess in the TOLB group.

Criticism 2—Use of a Fixed Dose of Tolbutamide

Many critics, both clinical and statistical, have pointed out quite correctly that the use of a drug in a clinically irrelevant manner seriously compromises the clinical utility of a therapeutic trial. The decision to use

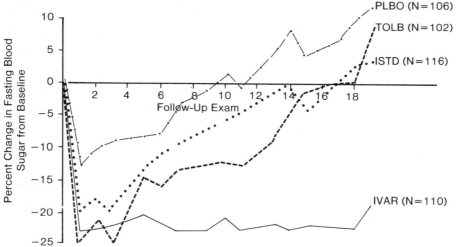

Figure 12.2.   Percent of Change in Fasting Blood Glucose Levels From Baseline to Each Follow-Up Examination for the Cohort of Patients Followed Through 19th Follow-Up Examination. (Adapted from University Group Diabetes Program. *Diabetes* 1970; 19 (Suppl 2):747–783.)

an invariate dose of TOLB rather than adjusting the dose to achieve optimal blood sugar control apparently stemmed from concerns about the mechanics of double-blinding a variable dose. In defense of the UGDP, 1.5 grams/day is a very typical dose and, as shown in Figure 12.2, reduced blood sugar by an average of 25% during the first year before gradually becoming less effective. Despite its relative lack of effectiveness in the later years of follow-up, TOLB-treated patients were always better controlled than PLBO-treated patients, despite which they experienced greater cardiovascular mortality. Thus, the selection of a fixed dose of TOLB may have been unwise, but it remains difficult to ascribe the mortality differences to this decision.

Criticism 3—Patients Who Stopped or Switched Treatments were Counted in Their Original Group

In any long-term trial of chronic therapy, a recurrent problem relates to the fact that therapy is often altered or stopped by the patient or the physician. If this occurs unequally in the groups being compared, it can influence the results. This occurred very frequently in the eight years of the UGDP trial, such that only 62% of subjects received all their assigned medication in 75% or more of their follow-up visits.

How can we examine the effect of this potential source of bias? If the excess mortality in the TOLB group resulted from deaths among individuals who received much less than the prescribed amounts of TOLB and/or were switched to other regimens, their removal from the analysis should diminish the mortality differences. Table 12.4 shows the cardiovascular mortality rates among those subjects who consistently received and took their assigned regimen. The mortality excess for cardiovascular deaths in the TOLB group, as compared with the PLBO group again increases rather than decreases.

Table 12.4
Number and Percentage of CVD Deaths in Patients with High Adherence to their Prescribed Regimen*

	PLBO	TOLB	ISTD	IVAR
High Adherers	143	151	119	96
CVD Deaths	5	22	11	3
CVD Death Rate (%)	3.5	14.6	9.2	3.1

* Adapted from Report of the Committee for the Assessment of Biometric Aspects of Controlled Trials of Hypoglycemic Agents. *JAMA* 1975; 231:583–608.

Criticism 4—Why Wasn't There an Increased Risk of Total Mortality?

Although the total mortality rate in the TOLB group exceeded all of the other groups, the difference between it and the PLBO group did not reach statistical significance. This is unfortunate because it leaves open the possibility that there was bias in the classification of deaths, i.e., that a death in the TOLB group was more likely to have been attributed to CVD than a death in the PLBO group. In fact, patients in the TOLB group who died received autopsies more often than those who died in other groups.

To protect against such a bias, the UGDP appointed a group who reviewed clinical material without knowledge of treatment and assigned the cause of death. Also, causes of death have been reviewed independently and a few changes were made which did not change the findings.

Although the all-cause mortality excess did not reach statistical significance, its change over time provides further evidence that it may have been meaningful. Figure 12.3 shows the cumulative mortality rates in the four groups. Two features of the curve support a toxic effect of TOLB. First, the early mortality in the TOLB group was low, suggesting that the randomization did not allocate a disproportionately large group of very sick patients to TOLB. Second, when the mortality excess did begin, after the fourth year of follow-up, it steadily increased.

Critics have shown that if the cumulative mortality is plotted until the end of the study, i.e., for the five years after TOLB was discontinued, the TOLB and PLBO curves move toward each other and coincide by 12 years of follow-up. They interpret this as evidence of peculiarities in the groups which evened out with time. An alternative and perhaps more

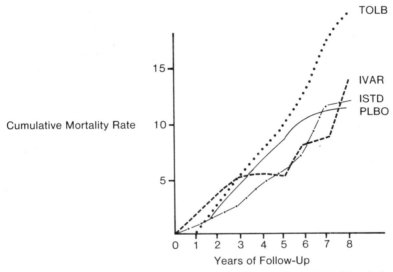

Figure 12.3. Cumulative Mortality Rates (All Causes) per 100 Population at Risk by Year of Follow-Up. (Adapted from University Group Diabetes Program. *Diabetes* 1970; 19 (Suppl 2):747–783.)

compelling explanation is that the removal of a toxic agent resulted in a slowing of the death rate in the TOLB group.

Criticism 5—Most of the Deaths Occurred in a Few Clinics

Patients were recruited by the 12 centers from very different sources ranging from community surveys to internal medicine clinics. Therefore, it is not surprising that the mortality rates differed among clinics such that 82% of the deaths occurred in five centers.

Some of the initial concern raised over the fact that a few clinics enrolled most of the patients who died resulted from a misunderstanding of the research design. These early critics overlooked the fact that randomization proceeded independently within each clinic so that if one clinic's patients had poorer prognoses, which proved to be true, that clinic's patients would be evenly distributed among the four treatment groups.

Nonetheless, because most of the deaths occurred in a few clinics, it raises the suspicion that there was something unique in those few clinics which could determine the overall results, particularly if the TOLB death rate excess were concentrated in one or two centers. Table 12.5 shows the CVD mortality rates by treatment group in the five clinics having the largest number of deaths. With the exception of one clinic (New York) all demonstrated a marked increase in CVD mortality in the TOLB group.

Criticism 6—More High Risk Subjects Were Enrolled in the TOLB Group

This is perhaps the most consequential of the criticisms leveled at the conclusion that TOLB is toxic. It suggests that the mortality differences resulted from differences in the risk characteristics of the groups at baseline rather than the treatments. In other words, the apparent toxic

Table 12.5
Cardiovascular Death Rates (%) by Clinic and Treatment Group*

Clinic	PLBO	TOLB	ISTD	IVAR
Cincinnati	8.7 (23)	31.8 (22)	16.7 (24)	19.0 (21)
Minneapolis	9.1 (22)	25.0 (24)	8.3 (24)	8.3 (24)
Williamson	4.3 (23)	13.6 (22)	8.7 (23)	12.5 (24)
Boston	6.7 (15)	23.5 (17)	6.3 (16)	6.7 (15)
New York	13.6 (22)	10.0 (20)	0 (21)	0 (22)

* Number of patients at risk in parentheses. Adapted from University Group Diabetes Program. *Diabetes* 1970; 19 (Suppl 2):785–830.

effect of TOLB is confounded by the greater initial CVD risk of the group receiving the drug.

Because many risk factors were measured at baseline, both the presence and the effect on mortality of baseline differences in risk factors can be evaluated. Table 12.6 shows the percentage of each group possessing various characteristics at baseline. The TOLB group is somewhat older than the PLBO group and contains higher proportions of patients with angina, digitalis use, elevated cholesterol, obesity, and arterial calcification. Because of these differences, it becomes imperative to control for any effect of these risk factor differences.

Table 12.7 illustrates one simple method of controlling for the effect of a single risk factor: dividing the groups into those who possess the risk factor and those who do not, then examining the effect of treatment separately in the two groups. Note that with very few exceptions, the TOLB group experienced greater CVD mortality both in the presence and in the absence of the risk factor.

However, looking at risk factors one at a time fails to account for the

Table 12.6

Percentage of Patients with Selected Baseline Risk Factors by Treatment Group*

	PLBO	TOLB	ISTD	IVAR
Age ≥55	41.5	48.0	46.2	46.1
Male	30.7	30.9	27.1	22.5
Non-White	49.8	47.1	51.0	40.7
Hypertension	36.8	30.2	30.9	28.1
History of Digitalis Use	4.5	7.6	5.8	5.0
History of Angina Pectoris	5.0	7.0	7.7	3.5
Significant ECG Abnormality	3.0	4.0	5.3	4.0
Cholesterol ≥300 mg/dl	8.6	15.1	16.4	13.4
Relative Body Weight ≥1.25	52.7	58.8	47.1	53.9
Arterial Calcification	14.3	19.7	17.2	15.9

* Data from: Seltzer HS. *Ann Rev Med*, 1980; 31:261–272. Adapted from University Group Diabetes Program. *Diabetes* 1970; 19(Suppl 2):785–830.

Table 12.7

CVD Death Rates (%) by Selected Baseline Risk Factors*

Baseline Risk Factors	PLBO	TOLB	ISTD	IVAR
Definite hypertension				
Absent	3.9	11.5	4.2	0.7
Present	6.8	13.3	10.9	19.6
History of digitalis use				
No	3.6	10.9	5.0	4.7
Yes	33.3	33.3	25.0	30.0
History of angina pectoris				
No	3.6	11.8	5.2	5.7
Yes	30.0	21.4	18.8	14.3
Significant ECG abnormality				
Absent	3.6	10.9	5.6	4.7
Present	33.3	50.0	18.2	37.5
Cholesterol				
<300 mg/dl	5.0	12.4	4.6	4.0
≥300 mg/dl	5.9	13.3	14.7	18.5
Relative body weight				
<1.25	7.2	15.5	6.7	9.6
≥1.25	2.8	10.8	5.8	2.7
Arterial calcification				
Absent	5.2	9.4	4.2	4.9
Present	13.8	25.6	25.7	22.6

* Adapted from University Group Diabetes Program. *Diabetes* 1970; 19 (Suppl):785–830.

well-known cumulative effect of several factors on the risk of CVD. Perhaps it is the combination of risk factors in the TOLB group which accounts for its greater CVD mortality. Table 12.8 shows the CVD mortality rates by treatment after dividing the patients according to the number of risk factors present at baseline. Although the TOLB group contains a greater percentage of patients with four or more risk factors, the excess risk of TOLB compared to PLBO is evident with all numbers of risk factors but one.

This simple method of combining risk factors ignores two other char-

Table 12.8
CVD Death Rates (%) by Number of Baseline Risk Factors and Treatment Group*

Number of Risk Factors	PLBO	TOLB	ISTD	IVAR
0	3.6 (28)	8.0 (25)	0.0 (22)	0.0 (15)
1	0.0 (60)	6.0 (50)	0.0 (62)	1.3 (76)
2	1.7 (59)	8.6 (58)	5.0 (60)	5.3 (57)
3	19.2 (26)	17.6 (34)	14.7 (34)	10.0 (30)
4+	16.7 (12)	31.8 (22)	29.4 (17)	55.6 (9)

* Number of patients in parentheses. Adapted from Cornfield J. *JAMA* 1971; 217:1676–1687.

Table 12.9
Observed and Expected CVD Deaths in the PLBO and TOLB Groups Where Probability of Death was Estimated from Risk Factors*

Probability of CVD Deaths	PLBO			TOLB		
	N	Observed	Expected	N	Observed	Expected
<0.0065	49	0	0.2	36	0	0.1
0.0065–0.0140	39	1	0.4	38	1	0.4
0.0141–0.0295	44	0	0.9	35	4	0.7
0.0296–0.0664	34	2	1.6	54	9	2.4
>0.0666	41	7	6.9	41	12	7.1
Total	205	10	10.0	204	26	10.7

* Data from Cornfield J. *JAMA* 1971; 217:1676–1687.

acteristics of CVD risk factors—they are not equally powerful and their joint effects are not simply additive. Using complex statistical techniques, risk factors can be combined to produce an overall prediction of the risk of CVD mortality for an individual. Cornfield applied such an approach, called a multiple logistic function risk estimation, to the PLBO and TOLB groups and divided them into categories of risk as shown in Table 12.9 (8). The risk equation predicted 10 CVD deaths in the PLBO group, exactly what was found; it predicted 10.7 CVD deaths in the TOLB group which was less than one-half of the 26 deaths which actually occurred. The observed TOLB deaths exceeded the expected number of deaths at almost all levels of risk.

The reader has probably noticed that none of these analyses of CVD risk factors includes consideration of cigarette smoking. Cigarette smoking was not assessed and the UGDP was roundly chastised for the omission. Is it possible that differences in the smoking characteristics of the TOLB and PLBO groups accounted for the mortality differences? As pointed out in Chapter 7, Cornfield addressed this question by assuming that the prevalence of smoking in the TOLB group was 20% higher than in the PLBO group (the likelihood of this occurrence is 1 in 50,000). Even in this extraordinary situation, one would expect only a 16% increase in CVD deaths, not the 160% increase actually observed.

Criticism 7—The Placebo Group Had a "Spuriously" Low Cardiovascular Mortality

A serious threat to the credibility of the UGDP study was created by the recent defection of one of its member institutions to the anti-UGDP camp. In a recent paper, this group argued that the best explanation for the apparent toxicity of TOLB rests with the peculiarly low CVD death rate in the PLBO group (5), a recurrent criticism over the years.

Those convinced that the PLBO group was peculiarly healthy point out that the mortality experience of the PLBO group was less than what is generally found.

This could have arisen because patients in the study as a whole had an unusually good prognosis; or because once in the study, patients with particularly low risks tended to be assigned to the PLBO group.

The fact that mortality in the PLBO group was somewhat less than that generally encountered by diabetics confirms an observation made in many randomized controlled clinical trials—that the untreated group tends to do quite well. This most probably reflects the careful selection of subjects for study. In the UGDP study, patients were excluded if their physician believed that they could not survive for five years. Table 12.9 provides further evidence that the PLBO group's mortality experience was not bizarre. A standard CVD risk equation precisely predicted the number of CVD deaths. In other words, the PLBO group's CVD mortality rate conformed to expectations based on its baseline characteristics. There is no evidence that the randomization scheme was willfully or accidentally violated so that it becomes a question of whether the findings were influenced by bad luck. If bad luck in the randomization accounted for the findings, the statistical tests applied tell us that the chance of that occurrence was five in 1000, which we can evaluate for ourselves. Moreover, Table 12.9 shows that the groups were of similar risk, at least for many of the known risk factors.

CONCLUSION

Clearly, the UGDP study was flawed (as are most, if not all, research endeavors). Some flaws, like a high degree of medication stopping and switching are the inescapable consequences of doing research on free-living human beings who are cared for by many different physicians over a long period of time. Other flaws, such as the use of a fixed dose of drugs, were conscious decisions made for sensible reasons. Other flaws, such as the failure to measure cigarette smoking, were unfortunate oversights.

The question is, however, whether these flaws could account for the findings indicating that Tolbutamide is cardiotoxic.

As we have tried to show from an examination of published data using clinical epidemiologic methods, corrections for these flaws or group differences did not reduce the CVD mortality excess of the TOLB group.

As indicated in Chapter 11, this by no means proves that TOLB is toxic. Rather, it simply makes bias a less likely explanation for the observed association between CVD death and TOLB in this study. No other human study has demonstrated this apparent toxicity and evidence from animal experimentation is inconclusive. Therefore, we are left with an observation which, although unsupported by corroborating evidence, seems to be sound and must, until new evidence arrives, enter into clinical decision-making.

On balance, the preceding analysis suggests that the textbook discussions of oral hypoglycemic agents quoted at the beginning of the chapter are factually correct but perhaps give more credence to the criticisms than is supported by the data. Of some concern is the statement that "in the elderly female . . ., the correction of her discomfort associated with

Table 12.10
CVD Death Rates in TOLB and PLBO Groups by Age and Sex*

	Men		Women	
	Age (years)		Age (years)	
	≤53(%)	>53(%)	≤53(%)	>53(%)
TOLB	5/26 (19.2)	6/37 (16.2)	1/71 (1.4)	14/70 (20.0)
PLBO	1/28 (3.6)	6/35 (17.1)	1/85 (1.2)	2/58 (3.4)

* Adapted from Kilo C, Miller JP, Williamson JR. *JAMA* 1980; 243:450–457.

the glycosuria may far outweigh the theoretical increased risk of sudden death as found in the UGDP study." It is not clear why the author singled out elderly females because, as illustrated in Table 12.10, it was among elderly females that the largest TOLB mortality excess was found.

We do not intend to demean a much-valued textbook but rather to illustrate a more general point about textbooks and review articles which summarize and interpret multiple sources of evidence. Such reviews introduce an additional element between the research findings and the reader—the reviewer. Many reviewers are skilled in the principles and techniques of human research design and analysis, but some who are also members in good standing in the academic community are not. Also, reviewers may or may not have preconceptions which color their interpretation and evaluation of the relevant research findings. Because most reviews do not reiterate the methods and findings in detail, so that the reader can make an independent judgment, the clinician must be particularly cautious in the use of these summary sources of clinical information.

To return to the patient, Ms. HC, we have reviewed the evidence, considered the criticism and now must choose a therapeutic approach.

Our decision will rest on our judgment as to the discomforts and risk which insulin therapy represents for this woman as opposed to the increased probability of premature death related to oral hypoglycemic treatment. Decisions about individual patients like Ms. HC remain a matter of clinical judgment, and clinical epidemiology is not synonymous with clinical judgment. Rather, like physical diagnosis, clinical epidemiology serves as another means of acquiring accurate, relevant clinical information which then must be thoughtfully considered in the context of the individual patient.

SUMMARY

The purpose of this chapter, and of the book as a whole, is to illustrate how the non-researcher can become an active participant in the critical analysis of an important piece of clinical research. In the example used, various experts have formulated and addressed the questions for us, and all that was required to follow their arguments was an understanding of sources of bias and some general methods for estimating their effect. Contrary to widespread opinion, such critical analysis rarely requires detailed knowledge of complex biostatistical formulae. Armed with an understanding of the strengths and weaknesses of various research designs and methods of clinical measurement, the clinical reader need not feel intimidated by the scientific literature, a feeling which no doubt contributes to the difficulty many clinicians have in trying to "keep up."

If we have convinced our readers that the busy clinician can independently and logically decide whether a set of clinical or research findings is useful or not, and that the process of deciding can be intellectually challenging and rewarding, then we have done justice to the contribution Clinical Epidemiology can make to the better care of patients.

References

1. University Group Diabetes Program. A study of the effects of hypoglycemic agents on vascular complications in patients with adult-onset diabetes: I. Design, methods and baseline results. *Diabetes*, 1970; 19 (suppl 2):747–783.
2. Schor S: The University Group Diabetes Program: A statistician looks at the mortality results. *JAMA*, 1971; 217:1671–1675.
3. Seltzer HS: A summary of criticisms of the findings and conclusions of the University Group Diabetes Program (UGDP). *Diabetes*, 1972; 21:976–979.
4. Feinstein AR: How good is the statistical evidence against oral hypoglycemic agents? *Adv Intern Med*, 1979; 24:71–95.
5. Kilo C, Miller JP, Williamson JR: The Achilles heel of the University Group Diabetes Program. *JAMA*, 1980; 243:450–457.
6. Seltzer HS: Efficacy and safety of oral hypoglycemic agents. *Ann Rev Med*, 1980; 31:261–272.
7. University Group Diabetes Program. A study of the effects of hypoglycemic agents on vascular complications in patients with adult-onset diabetes: II. Mortality results. *Diabetes*, 1970; 19 (suppl 2):785–830.
8. Cornfield J: The University Group Diabetes Program: A further statistical analysis of the mortality findings. *JAMA*, 1971; 217:1676–1687.
9. Report of the Committee for the Assessment of Biometric Aspects of Controlled Trials of Hypoglycemic Agents. *JAMA*, 1975; 231:583–608.

Index

Abnormality, 2, 15, 18, 31ff
Absolute risk, 102
Accuracy, 53
Adherence, 146
Agreement, 52
Allocation
  non-random, 137
  of treatment, 137
  random, 138
  stratified random, 139
Analysis of variance, 159
Anemia, 34
Angina pectoris, 14, 84
Antibiotics, 158
Anticoagulants, 136, 138
Antihypertensive agents, 144
"Art of medicine," 9, 21
Aspirin, 192
Associations
  reversible, 200, 201
  strength, 197
Assuming the worst, 122, 124
Asthma, 84
Attributable risk, 101, 102, 103, 104

Bacille-Calmette-Guérin, 13, 14
Bacteriuria, 172
Bayes' theorem, 53
Benefits, 14
Bias, 6–11, 13, 192
  assembly, 13, 118, 119
  case control studies, 178–183
  clinical trials, 133–145
  cohort studies, 118–121
  confounding, 6, 7, 13
  controlling, 121–125
  diagnostic tests, 52
  measurement, 6, 7, 8, 13, 121, 180, 193
  migration, 120
  potential, 118
  prevalence studies, 80–83
  publication, 145
  sampling, 11, 12, 109, 110
  selection, 6, 7, 8, 13, 120, 193
Biologic plausibility, 200, 201
Blinding, 141
Blood pressure, 9, 37, 42
Breast cancer, 112, 162, 178
Breast examination, 112

Cardiovascular disease, 120
Case control studies, 100, 171–183, 193
  advantages, 172
  bias in, 178–183
  versus cohort study, 173
  versus prevalence study, 176
Case finding, 67
Case, 81, 83
Case report: see Studies
Case series, 170
Cause, 2, 15, 80, 93, 95, 187, 201
  immutable, 188
  interaction, 189
  multiple, 188
  proximity, 190
  single, 188
  treatable, 188
Central tendency, 27, 28
Cervical cancer screening, 196, 197
Chance, 5, 6, 9, 10, 13, 145, 153, 193
Chi-square, 159
Cholecystography, 44, 46
Cholesterol, 35
Cigarette smoking, 102, 185, 199
Classification, 18
Clinical course, 109
Clinical epidemiology, 2, 5, 6
Clinical experience, 128
Clinical judgment, 217
Clinically important, 157
Clinical medicine, 4
Clinical questions, 1, 2, 16
Clinical research, 4
Clinical situation, 60
Clinical trials, 37, 131–151, 193
  bias in, 131–145
  explanatory, 140
  management, 140
  structure, 132
  uncontrolled, 133–136
Coherence, 201
Cohort, 96, 97, 115
Cohort studies, 97–100, 131, 179, 193
  concurrent, 98, 99
  historical, 98, 99
Commission on Chronic Illness, 84
Comparison group, 132
Comparisons, 122
  multiple, 164, 165
Compliance, 68, 69, 146

Confidence intervals, 156
Consent forms, 149
Consistency, 200, 201
Control group, 132, 179, 180
Controls
    concurrent, 136
    historical, 136
    non-concurrent, 136
Controversy, 183
Coronary bypass surgery, 123
Coronary care units, 136
Coronary drug project, 130
Coronary heart disease, 35, 38, 61, 98,
    121, 130, 144
Cost, 70
Cost benefit analysis, 14
Cost-effectiveness analysis, 14
Curricula, 5
Cut-off point, 33

Data, 18
"Data dredging," 165
Death, 3
Decile, 29
Decision analysis, 14
Decisions, 5, 14, 217
Demographic groups, 60
Design of human research, 5, 193
Destitution, 3
Diabetes, 48, 49, 204
Diagnoses, 2, 94
Diagnostic strategies, 15, 59–67
Diagnostic tests, 15, 41ff
    accuracy, 43–46
    bias in: see Bias, diagnostic tests
    multiple, 62, 65
    parallel, 62, 64, 66
    prevalence and, 53, 54, 59–62
    serial, 62, 63, 64, 66
Digoxin concentration, 56
Disability, 3
Discomfort, 3
Disease, 3
    duration of, 82, 83
    mechanism, 95, 128, 169, 190
    outcome of, 110, 111
Dispersion, 27, 29
Dissatisfaction, 3
    actual, 28
Distributions, 27
    Guassian, 29

normal: see Distributions, Guassian
    skewed, 28
Dose-response relationships, 198
Duodenal ulceration, 163
Duration of disease, 83

Ecological studies: see Studies, ecolog-
    ical
Effectiveness, 68, 145, 146
Efficacy, 68, 69, 145, 146
Electrocardiogram, 61
Electrocardiographic stress test, 60
Endometrial cancer, 173ff, 199
Epidemiology, 3, 4
Error
    alpha: see Error, type I
    beta: see Error, type II
    type I, 154, 155
    type II, 154, 155
Erythroleukemia, 171
Estrogens, 174, 175, 180, 199
Ethics, 148
Etiology: see Cause
Events, 3, 15
Evidence, 127
Exercise, 8, 120
Experiment, 95, 131, 132
Exposure, 92, 180

False negative, 43
False positive, 43
False positive rate, 49
Fibrinogen, $_{125}$I-labeled, 64
"Five D's," 3
Framingham study, 98, 121
Frequency, 2, 15, 75ff
Frequency distribution, 27

Gallstones, 44
Generalizability: see Validity, external
Gold standard: see Standard, gold
Gout, 36
"Grading" the evidence, 201

Halothane, 169
Hawthorne effect, 134
Hepatitis, 169
Hereditary spherocytosis, 109
Herpes Zoster, 129
Hodgkin's disease, 119

Holmes, Oliver Wendell, 185
Hyperparathyroidism, 32, 33
Hypertension, 37, 103, 143
   Veterans administration study of: *see*
      Veterans Administration
Hyperuricemia, 36
Hypotheses, 5, 127, 169
Hypothesis
   generating, 165
   testing, 165
   therapeutic, 127

Ideas, 127
Impedance plethysmography, 64
Incidence, 76, 77, 78, 79, 82, 83
Incidence density, 80
Independence, 65, 66
Information, 14
Informed consent, 148
Instrument, 22
Insulin, 205
Itching, 142

Journals, 203

Koch's postulates, 188

Labelling, 70, 71
Latency, 92, 173
Lead time, 68, 69
Life table analysis, 116
Longitudinal studies: *see* Cohort stud-
   ies
Louis, Pierre, 89
Lung cancer, 15, 102, 199

Mammography, 112
Matching, 122, 179
Mean, 28
Measurement, 20, 21
   hard, 21
   scales, 20
   soft, 21
Mechanisms of disease, 4, 5
Median, 28
Misclassification, 19
Mode, 28
Multiple comparisons, 164
Multiple sclerosis, 110
Multivariate adjustment, 122, 124

Myocardial infarction, 65, 108, 111, 129,
   130, 136–138, 192

Natural history, 15, 108
Normality, 2, 18

Observational studies, 95, 96, 131
Obsolescence, 131
Odds ratio, 176, 177, 201
Oliver Wendell Holmes, 185
Oral contraceptives, 103
Oral hypoglycemic agents, 204
"Origins of disease", 190
Outcome of disease, 2, 110, 112, 141
Over-matching, 180

"pα," 156
"pβ," 156
Pancreatic cancer, 157
Pancreatitis, 131
Pathogenetic mechanism, 187, 190
Pearson's product moment correlation,
   159
Percentile, 29
Periodic health examination, 67
Personal experience, 93
Person-year, 80
Pharyngitis, 47, 79, 88
Phenylketonuria, 78
Place, 132, 136
Placebo, 141, 205
Placebo effect, 142
Platelets, 192
Population, 4, 9, 32, 76, 85
   at risk, 78, 86
Population attributable fraction, 103
Population attributable risk, 103
Population risk, 101, 102, 103
Power, 160
Prediction, 94
Predictive value, 52–56
   negative, 46, 53
   positive, 46, 53, 54, 61
Prevalence, 46, 53, 54, 59, 76, 77, 78, 79,
   82, 83
Prevalence survey, 83, 176
Prevention, 95, 128
   primary, 128
   secondary, 128
Preventive health care, 67

Probabilities, 4, 106
Problem list, 19
Prognosis, 2, 15, 106, 107, 118
Prognostic factors, 107
Prospective studies: *see* Cohort studies
Prostatic acid phosphatase, 55
Prostatic cancer, 55
Publication, 145
Puerperal sepsis, 185
"P value," 156

"Quality control," 23
Quartile, 29

Randomization, 122, 125
Randomized controlled trial, 194, 201
Random variation: *see* Variation, random
Range, 29
Rates, 112
    case-fatality, 113
    five-year survival, 113
    incidence, 76
    prevalence, 76
    recurrence, 113
    remission, 113
    response, 113
    survival, 112
Receiver operator characteristic, 49, 50
Referral process, 59, 110
Regression to the mean, 37–39, 135
Relative risk, 101, 102, 176, 190, 201
    estimates, 177
Reliability, 22, 23
Research, 5
Research design, 150, 193
Reserpine, 178
Restriction, 121, 122
Retrospective, 171
Rheumatic complaint, 171
Rheumatoid arthritis, 79, 84, 86, 182
Risk, 2, 14, 15, 36, 87, 91, 92, 95, 98, 101–105, 107, 118
    attributable: *see* Attributable risk
    difference: *see* Attributable risk
    population: *see* Population risk
    ratio: *see* Relative risk
    relative: *see* Relative risk
"Risk factors," 91
ROC: *see* Receiver operator characteristic

Routine physical, 67
"Rule-in," 48
"Rule-out," 47

Sample, 9, 13, 24
    random, 85
    representative, 85
    size, 160
Sampling, 147
    fraction, 24
Scales
    interval, 20, 41, 42
    nominal, 20, 41, 42
    ordinal, 20, 41, 42
Scanning, 64
Screening, 67
    mass, 67
    recommendations, 72
    test criteria, 69–71
Seizures, 11, 12
Sensitivity, 46, 47, 48, 49, 51, 53, 55
Sickle-cell trait, 96
Significant difference, 157
Skewed: *see* Distributions
Spearman's rank correlation, 159
Specificity, 46, 47, 48, 49, 51, 53, 55
Spectrum of patients, 51
Standard deviation, 29
Standardization, 122
Standards
    gold, 43
    imperfect, 45
    objective, 45
"Statistically significant," 56, 156
Statistical tests, 154
Statistics, 5, 153
    inferential, 27, 155
Strata, 122, 123, 139
Stratification, 122, 123, 139
Stratified randomization, 139
Streptococcal pharyngitis, 75, 88
Student's t-test, 159
Studies
    case-control, 132, 171, 179, 201
    case reports, 169
    case series, 170
    cohort: *see* Cohort studies
    cross-sectional, 78
    ecological, 196
    experimental, 96, 132, *see also* Clinical trials

incidence: *see* Cohort studies
intervention, 132, *see also* Clinical trials
longitudinal: *see* Cohort studies
multi-center, 169
observational, 95, 96, 131
prevalence, 78, 176, 179
prospective: *see* Cohort studies
retrospective: *see* Case control studies
time series, 195, 201
Subgroups, 143, 144
Survival analysis, 114, 116
Survival cohorts, 99
Survival curve, 116–118
Systematic errors, 5, 6
Systemic lupus erythematosis, 135

Tampon, 186
Target population, 154
Temporal relationships, 195
Test of significance
one-tailed, 158, 159
two-tailed, 158, 159
Textbooks, 203
Thrombosis, deep vein, 63, 65
Time, 79, 80, 132, 136
Time series: *see* Studies, time series
Tolbutamide, 205
Toxic shock syndrome, 186, 195
Treatment, 2, 15, 127, 128
allocating, 137
Trial: *see* Clinical trials

Trial on antihypertensive agents, 37
True negative, 43
True positive, 43
Truth, 6, 43
T-test: *see* Student's t-test
Tuberculosis, 13, 14, 24, 190, 191

Uncertainty, 4
University Group Diabetes Program, 124, 204ff

Validity, 7, 21, 22, 26, 45, 132
external, 11, 13, 87
internal, 11, 12, 13, 130
Value judgments, 14
Variability, 161
Variation, 23
biologic, 23, 24, 25
effects, 26, 27
instrument, 23, 24
measurement, 23, 24
observer, 23, 24
random, 26, 31, 38, 153
sources of, 23–26
Venography, 63, 65
Ventricular premature depolarization, 24
Veterans administration, 12, 37, 144

"Web of causation," 188
"Worst case," 124

"Zero-time," 112